Investing in Health: Building a Stronger Public Healthcare System in India

Naviya

Table of Contents

Introduction

India has a pluralistic health system with a thriving private sector that is poorly regulated, and a public sector that is historically under-funded.[1, 2] While the federal government sets broad policies and programs for the public healthcare system, primary responsibility for health rests with the state governments – making the system extremely complex. As of 2015-16, India's total health expenditure was estimated to be 3.84% of its gross domestic product (GDP), while government health expenditure constituted less than one-third of the total health expenditure.[3] Though the private sector provided about 80% of outpatient and 60% of inpatient care[4], an estimated 86% of the spending to access private health care in the country was out-of-pocket expenditure – often leading to impoverishment in both rural and urban areas.[5, 6] Continued under-funding and neglect of the public health system had contributed to deep-rooted inequities within India's healthcare system – the burden of direct out-of-pocket expenditure increased much faster, from 1999-2000 through 2011-2012, for the poorest 20% among the socio-economically disadvantaged communities.[7] As of 2005, the differential in under-five mortality rate between the richest (27/1000) and poorest (85/1000) wealth quintiles was a striking 58 per 1,000 live births.[8] The National Commission on Macroeconomics and Health had noted that key factors adversely affecting the functioning of public health system included poor management of resources, centralized decision-making, low budgets, irregular supplies, large-scale absenteeism, absence of performance-based monitoring, and lack of transparency and accountability.[9] Indeed, decades of neglect had severely compromised the capacity of the district and sub-district level public health system to deliver basic and essential health care services.[10]

The public health system in Bihar, one of the poorest states in the country, is symbolic of most of these challenges. Bihar (vide **Figure (i)** below) is India's most densely populated state with 104 million people, 89% of whom live in rural areas.[11] The state has a three-tier public healthcare delivery system[12] according to the level of care mandated to be provided by the different health facilities – Level 1 facilities are village-level clinics that provide basic care services; Level 2 facilities are the primary health centers that are mandated to have the capacity to provide basic emergency obstetric and newborn care (BEmONC) services; while Level 3 health facilities refer to all higher institutions (above primary health centers) – community health centers, referral hospitals, sub-divisional hospitals, district hospitals, and medical colleges – that should be able to provide comprehensive emergency obstetric and newborn care (CEmONC) services.

The state of Bihar had experienced major governance paralysis between 1990 and 2005 which led to severe under-utilization of federal funds and stagnant economic growth, adversely affecting all social sector development programs including those on health and poverty.[13] As of 2005, Bihar ranked dismally on several key health indicators: highest fertility rate in the country (total fertility rate=4.0), second-highest in proportion of under-five children who were underweight-for-age (56%), and among the top-five states in terms of maternal (MMR=312/100,000 live births) and infant (IMR=62/1000 live births) mortality. Further, it was reported that only 22% of live births and 18% of all deaths received any medical attention at a health facility in the state, while only one-third of all children aged 12-23 months were fully immunized against six vaccine-preventable diseases.[14, 15]

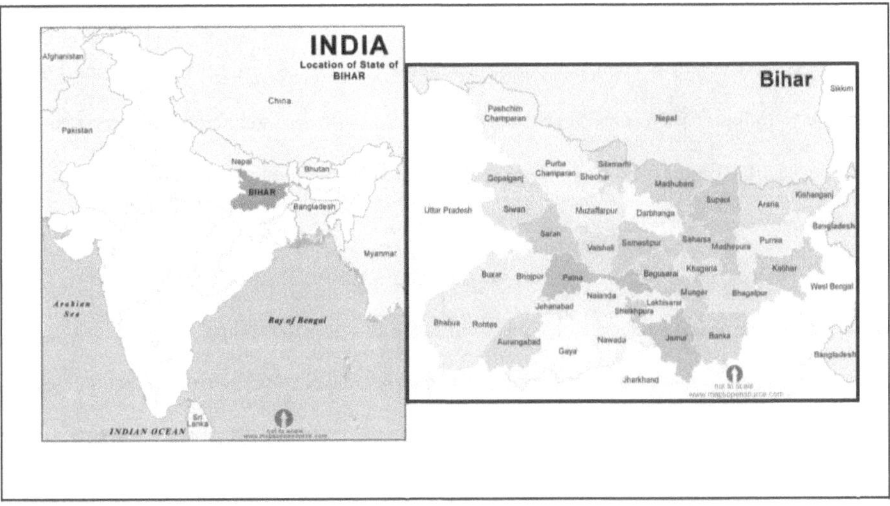

Figure (i): Maps showing location of the state of Bihar in India (left), and the 38 districts of the state (right) (Source: http://www.mapsopensource.com/)

With the change of political leadership in 2005 Bihar experienced considerable economic progress, and its GDP grew at an annual average of nearly 18% over the next decade.[16] Over the next five years Bihar's state health system demonstrated significant progress through increasing immunization coverage from 33% in 2005 to 67% in 2010 and institutional deliveries from 4% in 2006-07 to 50% in 2011-12.[16, 17] In this revitalized health environment, the Government of Bihar entered into a partnership with the Bill & Melinda Gates Foundation in 2010 to achieve accelerated progress in areas of maternal and child health, immunization, malnutrition, family planning and control of infectious diseases.[18]As part of this joint endeavour, the Integrated Family Health Initiative or IFHI (2011-2013) project was launched across eight programmatically-prioritized districts in the state, with CARE India being the lead implementation partner. The IFHI was a supply-side oriented program primarily concentrated on facility-based and outreach-based delivery of solutions, and aimed to increase the coverage and quality of life-saving, high-impact and cost-effective interventions, and improve the health, survival and nutrition of women, newborns and children during the first 1,000 days (conception to second birthday).[19] IFHI recorded commendable success stories like increasing home-visits by front-line health workers from 6% to 29%, improving early initiation of breast feeding from 39% to 59%, complementary feeding practices from 30% to 77%, and achieving 19% increase in providing counselling on family planning services (from 10% to 29%).[20]

However, IFHI was not really mandated to address the system-wide shortcomings in basic infrastructure and human resources that plagued Bihar's public health system. Through the insights gained during the three-year program implementation period, the Bihar government and its development partners realized that unless these system-wide shortcomings could be holistically addressed, much of the IFHI's successes would be unsustainable. For example, if there were no functional primary health centers that could ensure basic minimum care during labor, merely increasing antenatal home-visits by community health workers would make little difference in the overall maternal mortality numbers. There was 48% shortfall in the number of functional sub centers, 39% shortfall in PHCs and 91% shortfall in community health centers across the state, as well as 27% shortage in the required number of nursing staff at primary and community health centers.[21] Further, the overall lack of government ownership of the systems being put in-place by development partners was also noted as a cause of concern. It became evident that unless these fundamental system-wide gaps were addressed through state-level policy and planned health system strengthening efforts, a program like IFHI may not be able to reach its desired level of success.

Thus, in November, 2013 the Bihar government and its development partners realized that there was an urgent need to develop a health system strengthening approach to achieve sustainable improvement in population health outcomes – in other words, the IFHI approach needed

transformation. Hence, the Bihar Technical Support Program (BTSP) was established as a formal

structure for co-ownership of development goals between the state government, funding agencies

and implementation partners. Since 2014, while the programmatic focus remained on

reproductive, maternal, newborn, and child health (RMNCH) and nutritional outcomes, the

development agencies assisted the Government of Bihar to identify and strengthen health system

gaps in infrastructure, supply chain, human resources, and data-driven decision-making.[19] In

particular, CARE India (as the lead NGO partner providing techno-managerial assistance) was

entrusted with providing strategic and technical support at the state level, implementation, skill-

building and mentoring support at the district and block levels, and data collection and analysis

support at all levels. In order to design and implement data management systems that would

generate, analyze and disseminate data on community and facility level services at scale, CARE

India established an independent Concurrent Monitoring and Learning Unit, separate from its

implementation/ program management arm.

At the facility-level, the BTSP adopted a two-pronged strategy. On one hand, BTSP utilized

annual/ biennial comprehensive facility assessments(CFAs) conducted by the Concurrent

Monitoring and Learning Unit to identify and address gaps in facility-level infrastructure and

essential supplies, as well as rationalize the distribution of available health workforce. It was

hoped that this approach would help to improve the "facility readiness" (or, structural readiness)

of public health facilities to deliver health services. Simultaneously, the BTSP also conducted

on-site nurse mentoring programs to develop competency among the general nurse midwives

(GNM nurses) and auxiliary nurse midwives (ANM nurses) in providing BEmONC/ CEmONC

services. This intervention was known as the AMANAT program – an acronym for *Apaatkalin*

Matryitwa evam Nawjat Tatparta, which means emergency obstetric and newborn care (EmONC) service readiness.[22] AMANAT was targeted to improve the quality of care, and consequently, the "facility performance".

The aim of this book was to conduct an evidence-based assessment of the state-wide health system strengthening program in Bihar. Through three inter-linked papers, the book describes the evolution of the BTSP, analyzes the level of facility readiness achieved, and evaluates its association with facility performance. For this purpose, secondary analyses of quantitative data generated by the Concurrent Monitoring and Learning Unit of CARE India were conducted. Facility readiness was operationalized in terms of the availability of a number of facility-level characteristics including infrastructure, human resources, stock-in of functional equipment, consumables and drugs, referral transport system, laboratory services, and infection control and biomedical waste management practices. In the same context, facility performance was based on the direct observation of normal vaginal deliveries and newborn care provision, including management of immediate complications if needed, as well as labor room infection prevention practices.

The first paper (Chapter 1) describes the evolution of BTSP since 2014 – the context in which the Bihar government and its development partners realized the need for a health system strengthening approach (over narrower, vertical modalities) to bring about sustainable improvements in desired program areas. It looks into the governance mechanisms put in-place to foster co-ownership of program goals between the Bihar government and its development partners, aided by a strong system of data management, so that sustainability is built into this health system strengthening process. This was achieved through a structured, narrative review of the scientific and grey literature. Subsequently, the paper examines the initial progress made in a specific area of the overall health system strengthening process – the structural improvement of public health facilities (i.e., facility readiness) between 2015 and 2016, in terms of infrastructure, human resources, and supply chain. This part involved analysis of quantitative data generated through two rounds of CFAs conducted by CARE India in 2015 and 2016.

The second paper (Chapter 2) continues the quantitative assessment of facility readiness through utilizing comprehensive data generated by CARE India through the expanded CFAs conducted in 2017 and 2019. First, the paper conducts a comparative assessment of the status of facility readiness in public health facilities of Bihar between 2017 (at end of the first four years of BTSP) and 2019, and describes the continuation of progress or lack thereof. Second, the paper attempts to quantify facility readiness through the "facility-level maternal and newborn care (MNC) structural readiness score" – henceforth referred to as facility readiness score. An analysis of the trend in this score over time (2015, 2017 and 2019) across different districts and levels of health facilities in Bihar is also presented.

Thus, the first and second papers together examine the extent to which Bihar's public health facilities were structurally strengthened in terms of physical infrastructure, supplies and workforce by utilizing data from all four rounds of CFAs conducted till date. They seek to make an evidence-based argument in favour of undertaking exhaustive periodic exercises like the CFAs, as such assessments provide granular information regarding the structural gaps which affect functionality of public health facilities – and hence are key to needs assessment and bottom-up planning for health system strengthening.

The third paper (Chapter 3) asks the next logical question in a health system strengthening process – was facility readiness positively and significantly associated with facility performance? This is an important query, as it aims to provide evidence of synergistic progress, as envisioned under BTSP. First, the paper examines whether the facility-level performance changed, and this is accomplished by comparing the baseline (May-December, 2018) and endline (October-December, 2019) assessment data from the nurse-mentoring program, locally called AMANAT *Jyoti* (2018-present). Second, the paper assesses the association between facility readiness and endline facility performance in providing MNC services. This is accomplished by developing the baseline and endline "facility-level MNC performance scores" – henceforth referred to as facility performance scores, and examining the association of facility readiness score (based on CFA 2019 data) with the endline facility performance score. The findings help develop an in-depth understanding of the strengths of addressing infrastructural as well as quality issues as part of a holistic system-wide approach, while also pointing out the areas which require persistent attention.

The overarching purpose of this book is to present an evidence-based assessment of the facility-level interventions under BTSP – highlighting the strengths and challenges of developing the structural capacity of public health facilities while ensuring a minimum quality of services in an extremely resource-poor setting. The results seek to support the Bihar government and its development partners to better understand this health system strengthening process, encourage state health policymakers to become more engaged stakeholders, and guide purposeful allocation of resources to achieve efficient, equitable, and sustainable progress.

Chapter 1: Understanding the genesis of a health system strengthening program in Bihar, India (2014-present), and assessing the initial structural improvement of public health facilities between 2015 and 2016

1.1 Introduction

Bihar, located in the eastern part of India, is one of the eight designated socio-economically under-developed states – called the Empowered Action Group or EAG states.[23] As per the 2011 census, 89% of Bihar's 104 million population lived in rural areas, and the state recorded the highest population density (1102 persons/km^2), highest fertility rate (3.3 births/women), and lowest literacy rate (63.82%) in the country. An estimated 34% of the population lived below poverty level, with the proportion ranging between 47% and 72% in its most backward districts.[11, 24, 25] Combined these factors have historically affected health care and health outcomes.

The state had experienced major governance paralysis between 1990 and 2005 which led to severe under-utilization of federal funds and stagnant economic growth, adversely affecting all social sector development programs.[13] However, with change of leadership in 2005 the state's economic progress improved, and the government demonstrated intent to invest in the public health sector.[16] Consequently, the population below poverty level declined from 55% in 2005 to 24% in 2012,[25] while full immunization coverage among infants doubled from 33% in 2005 to 67% in 2010, and the proportion of institutional deliveries increased over 12-fold, from 4% in 2006-07 to 50% in 2011-12.[16, 17] Around the same time (in 2010), the Government of Bihar initiated a collaboration with the Bill & Melinda Gates Foundation – the *Ananya* partnership – to achieve accelerated progress in a number of priority areas in the health sector, with CARE India

as the lead implementation partner. Under this collaboration, the Integrated Family Health

Initiative (IFHI) was launched to deliver facility-based and outreach-based solutions targeting

maternal and newborn care, nutrition, immunization, family planning and control of infectious

diseases (elimination of visceral leishmaniasis).[18] The IFHI was implemented between 2011 and

2013 in eight programmatically-prioritized (high focus) districts of the state. However, through

these years of joint implementation, the government and its development partners recognized

that there were deep-rooted deficiencies within Bihar's public health system – and unless these

were addressed, it would be very difficult to achieve sustainable population health

improvements. The 2014-15 Rural Health Statistics report published by the Government of

India[21] revealed that the number of functional Primary Health Centers (PHCs) in Bihar was 60%,

and the number of Community Health Centers (CHCs, serving as first referral units) was 9% of

the numbers required as per population-based norms. The severe shortage of human resources for

health was also evident – there was 75% deficiency in the required number of public health

physicians, 27% deficiency in the required number of nursing staff, and about 80-90% deficiency

in the number of pharmacists and peripheral health workers at PHCs and CHCs.[21, 24] An analysis

of the 2014 National Sample Survey data[26] revealed that over 80% of both urban and rural

population in the state reportedly lacked access to public health services, and were compelled to

seek private health care even at significant out-of-pocket costs. Based on responses from

individuals who had recently suffered from some ailment, the principal barriers to utilizing

public health care were identified as the non-availability or poor quality of available necessary

services (for 64% rural and 58% urban population), physical distance of the facility from

residence (for 18% rural population) and long waiting times (for 30% urban population). It became evident that unless these fundamental system-wide gaps were addressed through state-level policy and planned health system strengthening (HSS) efforts, a program like IFHI may not be able to reach its desired level of success.

To address these systemic shortcomings, in November 2013 the Bihar Technical Support Program (BTSP) was launched to embark on a HSS effort to achieve improvements across reproductive, maternal, newborn and child health (RMNCH) and nutritional outcomes.[27, 28] It was envisaged that the development partners would work with the Bihar government to help initiate structural changes within the state public health system, specifically focusing on improving facility-level infrastructure, rationalizing the availability of human resources, and strengthening the supply chain for essential drugs, equipment and consumables. Thus, in essence, the HSS program in Bihar focused on what the Lancet Commission on high-quality health systems[29] described as the "foundations" of a health system: organizational and financial reforms in health governance, sustained investments in developing physical infrastructure of public health facilities (platforms), ensuring supply of essential medicines and equipment (tools), and building up a competent workforce – and all such changes being guided by robust data systems. The current paper describes the evolution of the state-wide HSS initiative in Bihar since 2014, based on the collective wisdom gathered by the state government and its development partners through the years of implementing facility-based and outreach-based programs. This was accomplished through a structured, narrative review of the scientific and grey literature. Subsequently, the paper attempts to assess the actual progress achieved within a specific domain of the overall HSS initiative – the structural improvement of public health facilities. This objective was addressed through measuring the tangible change in select facility-level characteristics (like availability of human resources and condition of the labor rooms in terms of infrastructure, functionality of equipment, supply of drugs and consumables), utilizing data generated through two rounds of Comprehensive Facility Assessments (CFAs) in 2015 and 2016 conducted by the Concurrent Measurement and Learning unit of CARE India. This data-based assessment also serves to facilitate a better understanding of the challenges in structurally improving the public health facilities of Bihar, given the policy-level reforms.

1.2 Methods

1.2.1 Review and synthesis of literature

The first part of this paper serves to establish the context in which the HSS efforts were initiated in November 2013, and highlights how the development partner(s) strived to work within Bihar's state health system. The content of this paper was achieved through a structured, narrative review of the scientific and grey literature that sought to address the following questions:

(1) What was the state of the public health system in Bihar leading up to 2010, when the Government of Bihar entered into a partnership (*Ananya*) with the Gates Foundation to address maternal and child health program outcomes?

(2) How did the experience from implementing the IFHI program between 2011 and 2013 across eight programmatically-prioritized districts in the state shape the evolution of the state-wide HSS program in 2014?

(3) What were the in-built governance mechanisms of this HSS program that facilitated its integration within the state health system and hoped to ensure sustainability?

(4) What were the specific mechanisms under this HSS initiative that were designed to address the foundational components (infrastructure, supply chain and workforce) of Bihar's public health system?

The mainstay of this review was based on examining the grey literature, especially the documents published by the Bihar Government and CARE India, the lead implementation partner in this HSS program. In particular, CARE India's 2014, 2016, 2017 and 2018 annual reports,[30-33] 2014-16 and 2019 impact reports,[34, 35] and working papers,[27, 36], along with the reports published by the state Health Department, Finance Department and the Bihar Development Mission[16, 17, 37] provided rich, contextual information. Further, data on Bihar's health system was obtained from the World Bank[25] and from Government of India publications, including the National Health Accounts Estimates for FY 2015-16[3], Sample Registration System Bulletins,[15] National Family Health Surveys (2005-06 and 2015-16)[14], and Rural Health Statistics (2014-15).[21] All these documents/ reports are freely available in the public domain from the cited sources. The review of scientific literature involved searching PubMed and Google Scholar for publications with combination of keywords like "Bihar" and "health"/ "health system"/ "*Ananya*"/ "Integrated Family Health Initiative"/ "Bihar Technical Support Program" between January 2000 and December 2020. The search resulted in identifying publications that highlighted the historical context as well as different components of the current program, and provided complementary support to the evidence generated through the grey literature review.

488 scientific publications and 47 grey literature documents (reports) were retrieved after discarding duplications. 416 scientific publications were excluded through title and abstract screening, as these focused on individual health programs (like malaria, tuberculosis) or on clinical interventions not relevant to the current paper. 72 full-text scientific publications and 47 reports were further assessed, and 58 were excluded as they did not address any of the 4 research questions. Hence, 31 scientific publications and 30 reports were included in the final literature

review. A detailed flow diagram of the process followed in retrieving, screening and including the scientific and grey literature has been provided in **Appendix A.**

Since this was a narrative review of literature with an objective of addressing the 4 specific research questions outlined above, the evidence synthesis was informed by these pre-defined themes (research questions). An inductive approach was applied to analyze this evidence and its implications, and thereby present a critical account of the evolution of this state-wide HSS initiative in Bihar.

1.2.2 The CFA methodology

To address the second objective, a secondary analysis of the quantitative data generated through two rounds of CFAs in 2015 and 2016 was conducted.

The CFAs were designed and implemented as serial cross-sectional assessments of public health facilities in all 534 blocks of the 38 districts in Bihar. A census was conducted of public health facilities in Bihar that had conducted a minimum of 100 deliveries in the year prior to the assessment – termed "functional" health facilities for the purpose of the assessment. Thus, all functional PHCs, CHCs and similar facilities like Referral Hospitals and Sub-divisional Hospitals (henceforth referred to as CHC-level facilities), as well as the District Hospitals (DHs) were included during each assessment. The 2015 CFA was conducted in April-June 2015 and covered 534 functional health facilities, while the 2016 CFA was conducted in July-August 2016 and involved 550 functional health facilities.

While PHCs are mandated to have the capacity to provide Basic Emergency Obstetric and Newborn Care (BEmONC) services, all other higher-level institutions are expected to be able to provide Comprehensive Emergency Obstetric and Newborn Care (CEmONC) services. However, in reality, not all CHC-level facilities in Bihar are capable of delivering CEmONC services, since they do not satisfy the WHO signal functions.[38] In fact, many sub-divisional hospitals can only provide BEmONC services. Hence, during the CFAs, the designation of health facilities as PHCs or CHC-level facilities was done based on their actual capability to provide BEmONC or CEmONC services respectively, and that did not always correspond to their government-mandated denomination. This led to some facilities of a 'higher' type being considered under a 'lower' type (for example some CHCs offering only BEmONC services were categorized as PHCs).

To facilitate the CFAs, CARE India's Concurrent Measurement and Learning unit developed a standardized questionnaire guided by Government of India's National Quality Assurance Standards guidelines and tools, and the Maternal and Newborn Health Toolkit.[39, 40] During the 2015 and 2016 assessments, data was collected on two domains – availability of human resources, and condition of the labor room in terms of infrastructure and supplies (drugs, consumables and equipment). The data collection was done by trained block-level "measurement, learning and evaluation" (MLE) coordinators who had been recruited as staff under the BTSP. Between 2-6 days of labor were required to complete the assessment at each health facility using paper-based tools. The assessment methods consisted of direct observation of infrastructure (condition of wall, floor, roof etc.) of the labor room, assessing functionality of related equipment, as well as the physical counting of drugs and consumables. The block-level MLE coordinators also examined data on the availability of medical officers (primary care physicians), specialist doctors (obstetrician & gynaecologist or OBGYN, anaesthesiologist, pediatrician and general surgeon), and nursing staff (general nurse midwives (GNM) and auxiliary nurse midwives (ANM)). To ensure the quality of the data being collected, random spot-checks were conducted by district-level MLE Officers for 15% of the facilities in each district.

1.2.3 Quantitative data analysis

The data generated through the 2015 and 2016 CFAs (available with the Concurrent Measurement and Learning unit of CARE India) was analyzed using STATA SE v.15[41], and presented as the number (percentage) of facilities, according to the type (PHCs, CHC-level facilities and DHs), which satisfied each assessment parameter. Thus, the results have been presented as binary responses (yes/no), like a facility having a functional equipment (or a medicine) or a facility with structural concerns like presence of cracks/ seepages in the walls of the labor room. The data on the availability of human resources was anlayzed in terms of the number (percentage) of health facilities (as per type) which reported availability of "adequate" number of healthcare providers for each specific cadre. The criteria for determining an "adequate" number of personnel for each category of healthcare workers at each type of facility was based on the 2012 revised Indian Public Health Standards[42], and the minimum (essential) number was considered for defining "adequacy". Hence, for PHCs, the availability of 1 medical officer was considered adequate, as was the presence of 3 staff nurses (includes both GNM and ANM nurses). For CHC-level facilities, the availability of at least 2 medical officers, 10 staff nurses, and 1 each of the 4 specialist physicians was considered adequate (separately for each cadre). For the DHs, the criteria included at least 11 medical officers, 45 staff nurses and 2 each of the 4 specialist physicians. For each cadre of healthcare workers, the number "available for service" was calculated as [(positions filled through regular recruitment + those on rotation duty or deputed-in (from other facilities) + contractual staff) - (staff on leave for more than 3 months

+ those deputed-out to other health facilities)]. The results hence depict the actual status of the healthcare workforce on the ground at the time of the assessment.

1.2.4 Ethical approval

The review of literature and the use of CFA data in this manuscript was determined as "not human subjects research" (under 45 CFR 46) by the Institutional Review Board at Columbia University, New York, USA (Protocol #IRB-AAAT1461, decision dated July 20, 2020). The data generated through the CFAs related to select facility-level characteristics like availability of human resources, and physical condition of the health facilities in terms of infrastructure, functionality of equipment, and supply of drugs and consumables. This data was retrospective, and also did not contain any individual-level identifiers (non-human subject data).

1.3 Results

1.3.1 Understanding the HSS program in Bihar

1.3.1.1 The historical context: state of the public health system in Bihar leading up to 2010, when the Government of Bihar entered into a partnership with the Gates Foundation

As discussed earlier, in 2005 Bihar had just emerged from nearly two-decades of social and political turmoil characterized by dysfunctional governance and a systematic collapse of law and order. The state faced severe economic stagnation, which adversely affected all social sector development programs including those addressing health and poverty.[13, 43, 44] Between 1997 and 2006, Bihar consistently recorded the lowest utilization rates for federal grants among the states in India. Over this period, nearly 23% of the federally allocated funds for the state was not withdrawn, and 36% of the transferred funds was not utilized.[37, 45] The state ranked dismally on several key health indicators (Sample Registration System and National Family Health Survey data for 2005): highest fertility rate in the country (4.0 births/women), second-highest in the proportion of under-five children who were underweight-for-age (56%), and among the top-five states in terms of maternal (312/100,000 live births) and infant (62/1000 live births) mortality. Further, it was reported that only 22% live births and 18% of all deaths received any medical attention at a health facility in the state, while only one-third of all children aged 12-23 months were fully immunized against six vaccine-preventable diseases.[14, 15]

With the change in leadership, the state-level GDP grew at nearly 10% between 2005 and 2015 (the fastest among low-income states in India), and the proportion of population below poverty sharply reduced from 55% in 2005 to 34% in 2012, mainly driven by reduction of poverty in the rural areas (from 56% to 34%) than urban areas (44% to 31%).[25] The government demonstrated strong intent to improve the ailing health sector, and garnered financial support through the Government of India's National Rural Health Mission (NRHM) which was launched in 2005.[43, 44] NRHM was India's first major supply-side reform program that aimed to provide comprehensive support to improve coverage, access and quality of care of the rural healthcare delivery system. The national program further prioritized the eight EAG states.[23] The Bihar government sought to take advantage of this landmark initiative, and achieved significant progress through expanding full immunization coverage among infants from 33% in 2005 to 67% in 2010, and increasing institutional deliveries from 4% in 2006-07 to 50% in 2011-12. It utilized NRHM financing mechanisms to address the critical shortage in human resources by appointing front-line workers (FLWs), including over 72,700 village-level community health workers (called accredited social health activists or ASHAs) and 10,000 ANMs by 2010. The state health governance structure was also remodeled as per the NRHM guidelines, through establishment of a state health society along with district-level branches to provide decentralized program management.[16, 17]**Panel 1.1** depicts the changes in key health financing and outcome indicators for Bihar between 2005-06 and 2015-16, and contrasts the latter with national-level data for 2015-16.

In this revitalized health environment, the Bihar government entered into a partnership with the Gates Foundation in 2010, called the "*Ananya*" program, to achieve accelerated progress in areas of maternal and child health, immunization, malnutrition, family planning and control of infectious diseases (mainly elimination of visceral leishmaniasis).[18] "*Ananya*" focussed on improving both demand and supply-side indicators through a judicious mixture of proven and innovative approaches, but addressing the larger health system issues was not a core target of this partnership.[16, 18, 43]

Panel 1.1: Bihar – key health financing and outcome indicators[3, 14-16, 25]

Indicators	Bihar		India, 2015-16
	2005-06	2015-16	
Contribution of Bihar in India's GDP (% share) [1]	2.35	3.02 (2013-14)	n/a
THE as % of state GDP [2]	n/a	6.5	3.84
Government health expenditure as % of THE [2]	n/a	19.1	30.63
Private out-of-pocket expenditure as % of THE [2]	n/a	79.9	60.59
Population below poverty line [3]	55%	34% (2012)	22% (2012)
Crude death rate [4]	8.1	6.2	6.5
Total fertility rate (children per woman) [4]	4	3.4	2.2
Maternal mortality ratio (MMR) [4]	312	165	130
Infant mortality rate (IMR) [5]	62	42	41
Under-five mortality rate [5]	85	58	50
Unmet need for contraception [5]	23.9	21.2	12.9
Mothers who had antenatal check-up in the first trimester (%) [5]	18.7	34.6	58.6
Mothers who had full antenatal care (%) [5]	4.2	3.3	21
Institutional births (%) [5]	19.9	63.8	78.9
Institutional births in public facility (%) [5]	3.5	47.6	52.1
Children under age 6 months exclusively breastfed (%) [5]	28	53.4	54.9
Children age 12-23 months fully immunized (BCG, measles, and 3 doses each of polio and DPT) (%) [5]	32.8	61.7	62
Children with diarrhea in the last 2 weeks who received oral rehydration salts (ORS) (%) [5]	20.9	45.2	50.6

Legends: GDP: gross domestic product; THE: total health expenditure

Sources of information: [1]Bihar Report Card 2015; [2]National Health Accounts Estimates for India FY 2015-16, Govt. of India; [3]Bihar - Poverty, Growth & Inequality, World Bank (2016); [4]Sample Registration System (SRS) Bulletins, Govt. of India; [5]National Family Health Survey (NFHS) 3 (2005-06) and 4 (2015-16), Govt. of India.

1.3.1.2 The transformation: experience from implementing the IFHI (2011 - 2013) program shaping the evolution of a state-wide HSS program in 2014

Under auspices of the *"Ananya"* program, the IFHI (2011-2013) was launched in 137 blocks of eight programmatically-prioritized districts – *Patna, Samastipur, Saharasa, Begusarai, Khagaria, Gopalganj, East Champaran* and *West Champaran*, with CARE India being the lead implementation partner. Working closely with Bihar government's health and nutritional (Integrated Child Development Services or ICDS) programs, the IFHI was mandated to develop and test evidence-based solutions that could be quickly scaled up to improve the health and wellbeing of pregnant women, mothers and children (i.e., covering pregnancy till 2 years after birth). These interventions were both facility-based and outreach-based, and targeted improvement of outcomes across five core areas – maternal and newborn care, nutrition, immunization and family planning.[46]

The IFHI implemented a number of evidence-based cross-cutting solutions to generate demand for services, as well as to improve the quality of service provision. For example, the FLWs were trained and utilized to generate awareness among target beneficiaries on the entire range of family health services, from better birth preparedness and registering pregnancies to ensuring full immunization coverage. Simultaneously, facility-driven quality improvement initiatives and nurse mentoring programs were introduced to improve the quality of perinatal service provision.[46-48] A number of innovative solutions were also pilot-tested for future scale-up, including mobile-based apps for FLWs and interventions to foster team-based approaches. The FLWs were trained to use an app (developed through the CARE-Dimagi partnership) which would allow them to efficiently and transparently perform client engagement activities like scheduling regular follow-up and completing necessary documentation. Further, sub-centre (village-level clinic) based platforms were created to enable the FLWs to discuss their achievements and obstacles, and be provided with structured supervision. Such platforms also offered the scope to launch a "team-based goals and incentives" program under which the entire FLW team at a sub-centre would be rewarded (non-monetary incentives) if the clinic achieved a set of pre-determined targets.[46, 48, 49] Finally, the IFHI ushered in systematic progress towards data-driven program management – by creating tools for health facility assessments, conducting direct observation of deliveries, clinical reviews and quality improvement meetings at health facilities, and implementing longitudinal and periodic cross-sectional surveys to evaluate interventions.[46, 48]

These evidence-based and innovative interventions contributed to some commendable success stories. Home-visits by FLWs increased from 29% to 62% during the last trimester (at least two visits), and from 6% to 29% during the first week post-delivery (at least three visits). Improvement in early initiation of breastfeeding (from 39% to 59%) as well as age-appropriate complementary feeding in terms of both quantity and frequency (from 30% to 77%) were observed following counselling by the FLWs on newborn care and feeding practices during their visits.[48, 50-52] The mobile-based intervention among FLWs helped them plan and execute these home visits. Data entry into the central server was real-time, as opposed to a mean 72-day lag for the paper-based system.[53, 54] There were indications that the team-based incentive program facilitated better quality of interactions between FLWs and their clients, especially in delivering advice on cord care, breastfeeding, complementary feeding, and family planning. Major improvements were also noted in terms of FLW team-coordination, self-reported job satisfaction, perception of empowerment, and satisfaction from public appreciation of their work.[55, 56]Following the nurse mentoring initiative, described in details elsewhere [57, 58], increased positive "labor practice indicators" like assessing vital signs, providing perineal support during delivery of the fetal head, administering uterotonic after birth, and adhering to infection control practices were noted.[58] Additionally, improved newborn-specific good clinical practices like placing the newborn on mother's abdomen after birth, cleaning the eyes with sterile gauze, ensuring skin-to-skin care, and helping the mothers to initiate breastfeeding were also observed.[57]

While the IFHI demonstrated that significant improvement in target areas could be achieved through supporting the FLWs and developing competency among the nursing cadre, the quality of services delivered (and hence the outcomes) remained critically dependent on the functionality of health clinics. In other words, this success was reliant on the presence of physical infrastructure, supply of essential drugs and equipment, and of course, availability of skilled providers. Over the three-year IFHI implementation period, the Bihar government and its development partners recognized that unless the shortcomings in these areas could be addressed, it would be very difficult to achieve sustainable population health improvements.[27, 28] As discussed previously, nearly 40% PHCs and 90% CHCs across the state were not providing necessary clinical services, handicapped by acute shortages in all levels of healthcare personnel, lack of ambulances, and insufficient availability of drugs, consumables, and medical equipment. These system-wide deficiencies directly affected the quality of clinical care services that could be provided.[21, 46] The IFHI program leadership hence perceived the need to adopt a HSS approach towards addressing these priorities, along with the critical importance of transferring ownership to the state health system.[43]

These realizations motivated efforts to broaden the scope of the *Ananya* program to address system-wide bottlenecks through state-level policy and planned HSS efforts, and led to the formation of the Bihar Technical Support Unit (TSU) in November 2013. The TSU was conceived as a formal structure for co-ownership of development goals between the state government (Health and Social Welfare Departments), funding agencies, and the implementation partners, with CARE India providing leadership in its formation and operationalization.While the overall focus remained on achieving improvement across RMNCH and nutritional outcomes, the development agencies were mandated to provide technical and implementation support to the Government of Bihar to adopt an HSS approach towards meeting the targets.[27, 28]The new program was designed to serve all 534 blocks in 38 districts of the state, and was thus mandated to be responsive to the health needs and outcomes for 2.7 million pregnant women and 2.55 million births/year, in contrast to 0.9 million pregnant women and 0.85 million births/year during the IFHI phase. Intervention support was now required for 180,000 FLWs (up from 46,000) and 25,000 nursing cadre (up from 5,000) over the course of the program.[28, 43] At the same time, it is important to note that the IFHI and BTSP (Bihar Technical Support Program) did not exactly share a pilot-and-scale up relationship. The IFHI phase was primarily about the development partners leading the implementation of evidence-based and innovative solutions through intensive efforts. On the other hand, the TSU mode of approach was really concerned about gradually transferring the ownership of health system strengthening efforts to the Bihar government – with appropriate modifications of the interventions, and the recognition that this process would be challenging. **Figure 1.1** presents a summary timeline of the origin and progress of this HSS program in Bihar.

This revised approach was greatly incentivized by the launch of the national RMNCH+A (RMNCH and adolescent health) program in January 2013. As a key component of NRHM, the RMNCH+A program aimed to establish a "continuum of care" for target beneficiaries by addressing obstacles in accessing and utilizing integrated healthcare services at both facility and community (home-based care) levels. The newly-conceived state-wide HSS program was built on the principles of the national RMNCH+A program, and this linkage further enabled the state government to leverage additional funds for its 10 most under-resourced and under-developed districts which were recognized as high-priority areas by the Government of India.[59-61] The HSS approach was also supportive of the Bihar government's (the then) newly launched Mission *Manav Vikas* (Human Development) which pledged to bring about holistic improvement in the quality of life of the citizens through integrated implementation of programs by the Departments of Health, Education and Social Welfare, among others.[62]

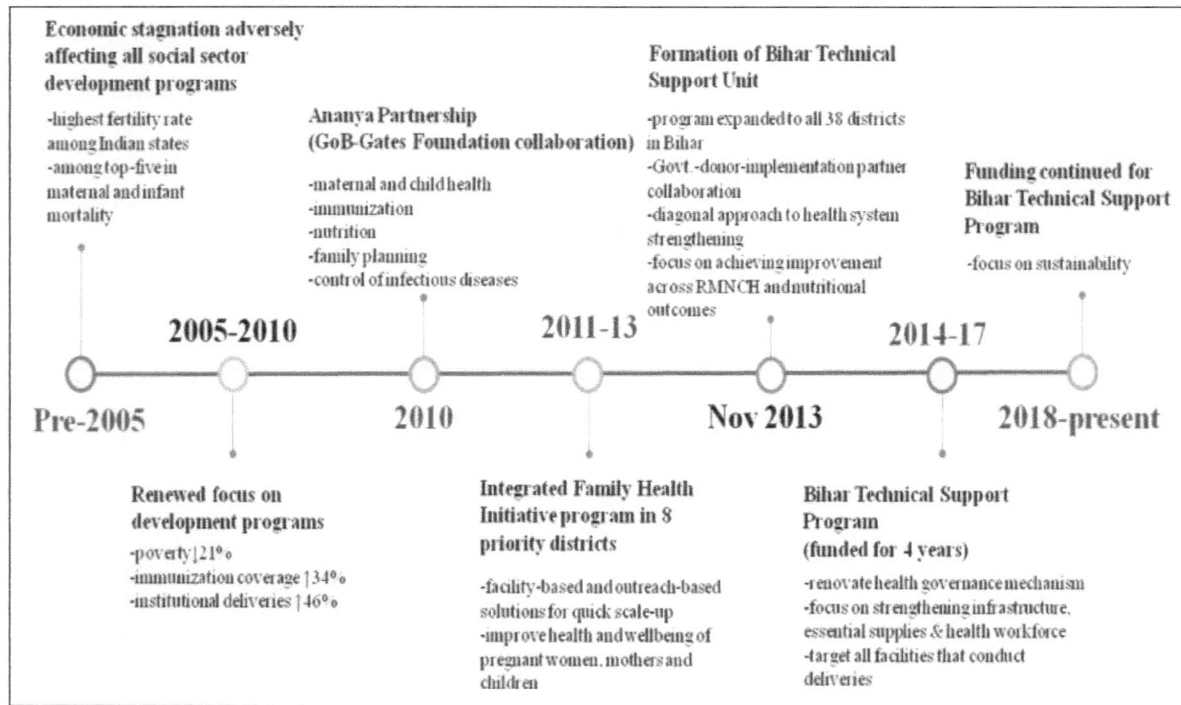

Figure 1.1 : Timeline of origin and progress of the health system strengthening program in Bihar
Legends: GoB: Government of Bihar, RMNCH: reproductive, maternal, newborn and child health

*1.3.1.3 Re-thinking health governance: in-built governance mechanisms of the HSS program to
facilitate integration within the state health system*

Under the TSU mode of operation, 4 inter-linked domains were targeted: (i) capacity building
within the state health system, focusing on improving public health leadership and managerial
skills to develop a culture of accountability towards achieving program goals; (ii) building
technical and managerial skills at the local levels to deliver on outreach and facility-based
programs; (iii) developing a system to generate, analyze and use data for continuous program
monitoring (keeping the focus on outcomes) as well as informing policy decisions; and (iv)
identifying and addressing the system- and policy-level barriers for better implementation of
RMNCH and nutritional interventions.[27] These activities ensued under the BTSP, and **Panel 1.2**
provides a broad overview of the 4 domains.

Panel 1.2: The domains for health system strengthening targeted under the Bihar Technical Support Program

Focus area 1: To develop leadership within the state health system and promote accountability in achieving program goals (focus on outcomes)

Key areas for action:
1. Enable the state/ district/ block health leadership to independently conduct monthly planning and review meetings and accordingly initiate improvement measures
2. Drive government ownership to implement solutions and take responsibility for outcomes
3. Institutionalize the delivery of techno-managerial inputs by development partners

Focus area 2: Building technical and managerial skills to deliver on outreach and facility-based programs

Key areas for action:
1. Systematically mentor district and block-level managers to implement various solution levers
2. Initiate on-site clinical mentoring of health care providers (focus on nurse mentoring)
3. Standardize and establish regular supportive supervisory mechanisms and quality improvement processes
4. Promote the use of information, communication and technology (ICT) to improve efficiency
5. Support improving the implementation of existing interventions

Focus area 3: To promote the use of data, and establish mechanisms for accountability

Key areas for action:
1. Promote the use of data dashboards to conduct evidence-based monitoring of progress
2. Provide supportive supervision at all levels of the state health system to conduct concurrent monitoring
3. Develop and implement tools and processes for focused supervision
4. Integrate "Concurrent Measurement and Learning" into the government system
5. Establish mechanisms to facilitate community feedback

Focus area 4: To address and overcome system- and policy-level barriers

Key areas for action:
1. Support the rationalization of human resources deployment and expansion
2. Track and support the stock-in of essential commodities at the facility level
3. Plan and implement new incentive-based approaches/schemes
4. Support expediting government-to-person payments (transferring cash assistance)
5. Stewardship of the private sector

To address the above mandate, it became necessary for the BTSP to develop a novel structure of health governance that would be deeply embedded within the state health system. **Figure 1.2** presents a schematic depiction of this governance mechanism. A state-level RMNCH Unit, in sync with Government of India's RMNCH+A program requirement, was established to usher greater synchronization between BTSP and the state Health Department, and to provide technical leadership on system strengthening, capacity building, and ensuring the quality of care. It was subsequently renamed as the State Resource Unit (SRU). Concurrently, a Nutrition Strategy Team (NST, coordinating with the ICDS program run by the state Social Welfare Department) was also constituted at the state level to ensure better implementation of nutritional schemes targeting reproductive-age women and children below six years of age, and to coordinate with the SRU. These two institutional mechanisms were expected to bring about greater efficiency and accountability within the state health system, and provide strategic and technical support to the state leadership to help push reforms in a top-down mode. The SRU was expanded to include both public policymakers and experts from partner organizations (including CARE, Govt. of UK's Department for International Development (DFID), Norway India Partnership Initiative (NIPI), UNICEF, and UNFPA), and was authorized to govern the implementation of several inter-related development programs in health and nutrition, each chaired by a team leader. To match the administrative structure at the district levels, District Resource Units (DRUs) were established in all 38 districts and staffed with a Team Lead and 4 program officers in each district - 3 District Technical Officers (for strengthening health facilities, managing outreach and nutrition programs, managing visceral leishmaniasis elimination program), and 1 District Monitoring and Evaluation Officer. As the lead partner in the TSU, CARE India followed through this structure till the block level, employing a block manager to interact with the local government, a block MLE coordinator to collect and manage data, and another block coordinator to work on the elimination program. This ensured that even at the block level, state-employed health care providers and FLWs would receive mentoring and support from partner agencies, thereby laying the foundation for both vertical and horizontal integration between the TSU and the state health system. Finally, a strategic program management team (SPMT) comprising of experienced technical leaders from different agencies was entrusted with conducting strategic analysis for and providing support to the SRU and DRUs.[27, 28, 30, 31, 34, 63] Moving forward, some potential challenges for the SPMT were likely to include maintaining real-time ground-level coordination with the government and BTSP district teams, and developing specific strategic plans for each district which would be aligned with the overall TSU strategy and goals.

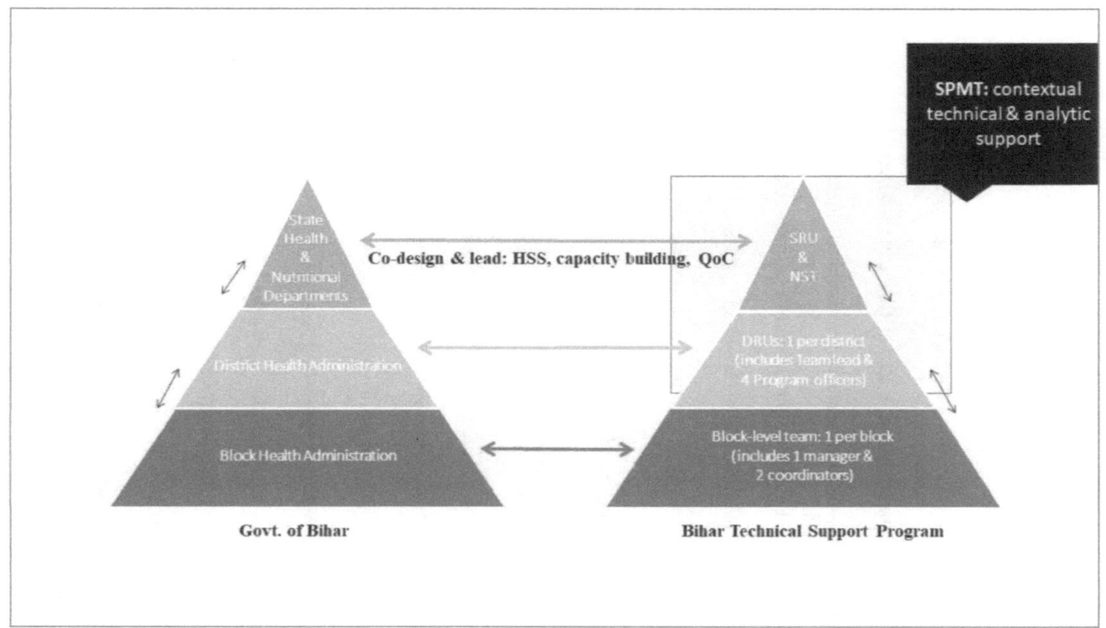

Figure 1.2: The health governance structure under the Bihar Technical Support Program

Legends: SPMT: Strategic Program Management Team; HSS: health system strengthening; QoC: quality of care; SRU: State Resource Unit; NST: Nutrition Strategy Team; DRU: District Resource Unit

Note: The bi-directional arrows between induvial levels within the Government system and the Bihar Technical Support Program indicate the bi-directional flow of information, resources and instructions. The connecting lines at a particular level between the Government system and the Bihar Technical Support Program indicate synchronized planning, implementation and monitoring.

1.3.1.4 Addressing the foundational components of Bihar's public health system: mechanisms to address gaps in infrastructure, supply chain and workforce

While the TSU approach brought together a large number of development programs on a common, coordinated platform, the key motivation behind its conception was to strengthen Bihar's public health system through identifying and addressing the foundational gaps, while also supporting the government in better management of financial resources.[63]

Identifying shortcomings in the physical infrastructure of public health facilities as well as maintaining a database on the actual availability of essential supplies like consumables, medicines, and equipment at the health facilities were identified as key challenges by the TSU. Consequently, the BTSP invested heavily in conducting expansive annual facility-level assessments (CFAs) covering all public health facilities in Bihar that conducted deliveries.[27, 28] It was envisaged that this data would directly help the Health Department to target its supply-side budget more efficiently through established institutional mechanisms like the Bihar Medical Services & Infrastructure Corporation Limited.[63, 64] The BTSP also attempted certain innovative approaches at the local level that could address supply-chain shortcomings while avoiding the long-drawn bureaucratic processes. These included, entrusting government-empaneled vendors to directly manage inventory and avoid stock-outs of drugs and consumables at the health facilities; training district-level officials to efficiently use the Logistics Management Information System to assess and replenish stocks from the state warehouses; and utilizing the FLWs to identify blood-donation camps and maintain a list of locally-available donors to address the periodic non-availability of blood products at the blood banks.[32, 33, 65, 66]

In order to address the critical shortage of trained manpower, the TSU prioritized providing technical assistance to the Health Department to rationalize its process of human resources management based on the urgent, unmet need at different levels of health facilities.[63]For example, specialist physician positions were first filled at the DHs, and subsequently at the Referral Hospitals and Sub-divisional Hospitals. The physicians who performed state or district-level administrative duties (e.g., chief medical officer of a district, malaria program officer) were no longer burdened with additional clinical rosters; while the process of inter-district transfers was restricted to only filling long-standing critical vacancies. Equally significant was the emphasis on developing competence among the nursing cadre in Bihar in order to address the quality of service provision. During the IFHI phase, CARE India had initiated a "mobile nurse mentoring team" (MNMT) program across 80 public health facilities in the eight programmatically prioritized districts to develop competency among nurses posted in the labor rooms. Under the BTSP, MNMT initiative evolved into the *AMANAT Buniyadi* (training to develop competency in providing BEmONC services) and *AMANAT Vyapak* (CEmONC services) programs. Under these two initiatives, expert nurse mentors from different reputed institutions in India were contracted to improve quality of service delivery through training Bihar government's ANM and GNM nursing cadres. Between 2014 and 2017, 320 additional public health facilities were covered, imparting training to about 3500 nursing staff. Since 2018, as the focus shifted towards sustainability, previously-trained government nurses with demonstrated professional efficiency were screened and selected as mentors for the next phase training of the nursing cadre (*AMANAT Jyoti*). The idea was to utilize the existing capacity within Bihar's public health system to train unskilled providers and ensure continuous capacity building of providers posted in labour room. The mentoring program was gradually expanded to cover Special Newborn Care Units (SNCUs) and obstetric operating rooms as well.[32, 43, 67-70]

Finally, building a robust information management system was identified as the basis of this HSS program. Consequently, a structurally embedded but functionally independent Concurrent Measurement and Learning unit was established by CARE India. This unit was mandated to design and implement data generation, management and analytics systems that would generate, analyze and disseminate data on community- and facility-level services at scale. Further, the unit was also entrusted to make this data available to public health officials at all levels in user-friendly formats to enable better decision making, while also monitoring and evaluating the innovations and approaches to enhance program learning.[28]To improve data-driven program monitoring and decision-making, a central data repository – the Health System Progress Tracker system – was created from all data sources across the state health system. This repository pooled data from the routine health management information system (for RMNCH indicators), the innovative android-based *Darpan/ Darpan Plus* app (for facility-level infrastructure and human resources data), as well as facility-level data on the indicators for supportive supervision which was being provided as part of BTSP (included data on OPD, maternal and neonatal services).[71-73] Simultaneously, there was a push towards using this data-based dashboard for conducting program reviews at the state, district or block levels through training of government staff and creation of a number of review forums like the district-level RMNCH task force meetings. It was hoped that these steps would contribute towards building a culture of accountability and using the program data.[63]

1.3.2 Examining progress in the structural improvement of public health facilities: 2015 and 2016 CFAs

While the earlier sections of this manuscript trace the genesis of the BTSP and describe key policies with regard to improving the foundational components of Bihar's public health system, the results from the CFAs conducted in 2015 and 2016 (presented below) help to quantitatively assess the impact of this HSS process on the functionality of public health facilities through the initial years.

During CFA 2015, a total of 534 functional health facilities were assessed, including 405 PHCs, 95 CHC-level facilities, and 34 DHs. On the other hand, CFA 2016 involved 550 functional health facilities including 420 PHCs, 96 CHC-level facilities, and 34 DHs. Six districts during the 2015 assessment were found to have no functional CHC-level facilities, but this gap was addressed in 3 of these districts by 2016. The DHs in *Darbhanga, Patna,* and *West Champaran* districts did not participate during either assessment, while *Purnia* participated only during 2016, and *Saharsa* only during the 2015 assessment. **Table 1.1** depicts the detailed district-wide breakdown of the assessed health facilities (according to level) during the 2015 and 2016 CFAs.

Table 1.1: Distribution of the assessed health facilities, CFA 2015 and CFA 2016

Sl. No.	Districts of Bihar	CFA 2015				CFA 2016				Change in total #facilities (2015 - 2016)
		PHC	CHC-level facilities	DH	Total	PHC	CHC-level facilities	DH	Total	
1	ARARIA	5	3	1	9	5	3	1	9	0
2	ARWAL	5	0	1	6	5	0	1	6	0
3	AURANGABAD	8	3	1	12	6	6	1	13	1
4	BANKA	7	3	1	11	7	3	1	11	0
5	BEGUSARAI	14	3	1	18	16	2	1	19	1
6	BHAGALPUR	10	5	1	16	11	5	1	17	1
7	BHOJPUR	11	4	1	16	11	4	1	16	0
8	BUXAR	8	1	1	10	9	1	1	11	1
9	DARBHANGA	14	6	0	20	17	3	0	20	0
10	EAST CHAMPARAN	16	4	1	21	19	3	1	23	2
11	GAYA	19	4	1	24	22	2	1	25	1
12	GOPALGANJ	9	4	1	14	9	4	1	14	0
13	JAMUI	6	3	1	10	6	3	1	10	0
14	JEHANABAD	6	2	1	9	7	2	1	10	1
15	KAIMUR	6	3	1	10	7	3	1	11	1
16	KATIHAR	13	3	1	17	13	3	1	17	0
17	KHAGARIA	5	1	1	7	5	1	1	7	0
18	KISHANGANJ	7	1	1	9	7	1	1	9	0
19	LAKHISARAI	4	1	1	6	4	1	1	6	0
20	MADHEPURA	13	0	1	14	13	0	1	14	0
21	MADHUBANI	18	2	1	21	18	3	1	22	1
22	MUNGER	7	1	1	9	7	1	1	9	0
23	MUZAFFARPUR	14	1	1	16	14	1	1	16	0

Continued

Sl. No.	Districts of Bihar	CFA 2015				CFA 2016				Change in total #facilities (2015 - 2016)
		PHC	CHC-level facilities	DH	Total	PHC	CHC-level facilities	DH	Total	
24	NALANDA	17	2	1	20	17	2	1	20	0
25	NAWADA	13	0	1	14	12	1	1	14	0
26	PATNA	19	7	0	26	19	7	0	26	0
27	PURNIA	6	3	0	9	9	4	1	14	5
28	ROHTAS	14	4	1	19	15	3	1	19	0
29	SAHARSA	9	0	1	10	8	1	0*	9	-1
30	SAMASTIPUR	16	4	1	21	16	4	1	21	0
31	SARAN	15	4	1	20	15	4	1	20	0
32	SHEIKHPURA	4	1	1	6	4	1	1	6	0
33	SHEOHAR	3	0	1	4	3	0	1	4	0
34	SITAMARHI	16	0	1	17	16	1	1	18	1
35	SIWAN	13	3	1	17	13	4	1	18	1
36	SUPAUL	8	2	1	11	8	2	1	11	0
37	VAISHALI	13	4	1	18	13	4	1	18	0
38	WEST CHAMPARAN	14	3	0	17	14	3	0	17	0
	TOTAL	405	95	34	534	420	96	34	550	16

Legends: CFA: comprehensive facility assessment; PHC: primary health center; CHC: community health center; DH: district hospital

1.3.2.1 Labor room – physical condition, equipment, drugs, and consumables

Tables 1.2 and **1.3** present results from the detailed assessment of the physical condition of labor rooms, and availability of functional equipment, medicines, and consumables, presented in terms of the number (percentage) of health facilities per level (PHC, CHC-level, DH) with the presence or absence of each parameter.

At least 96% of the assessed facilities in any category had designated labor rooms and at least 87% had designated newborn care corners (NBCCs) during CFA 2015, and this further improved over the next year. However, more significant was the marked increase in the proportion of health facilities which ensured that these NBCCs were located within the labor rooms (increase by 13 percentage-points among PHCs, 17 percentage-points among CHC-level facilities, 33 percentage-points among DHs). Across the board, the physical condition of the facilities in terms of cracks and seepage being reported from walls and/or roofs deteriorated between CFA 2015 and 2016. On the other hand, almost all facilities recorded availability of power back-up systems for labor rooms during both assessments, and remarkably improved the availability of elbow taps at hand-washing stations (at least increased 15 percentage-points in any category) over the one-year period.

The availability of all essential equipment (for which data was collected) improved among all types of health facilities between these two assessments. For example, by 2016, functional radiant warmers were available in 74% PHCs (increased 6 percentage-points), 84% CHC-level facilities (increased 10 percentage-points) and 91% DHs (increased 21 percentage-points); autoclave machines were available in 86% PHCs (increased 54 percentage-points), 92% CHC-level facilities (increased 56 percentage-points) and 94% DHs (increased 47 percentage-points); and neonatal oxygen masks were available in 93% PHCs (increased 39 percentage-points), 93%

CHC-level facilities (increased 35 percentage-points) and 94% DHs (increased 26 percentage-points). Varying levels of improvement were also noted for the availability of functional cord clamps, mucous extractors, newborn weighing machines, artificial manual breathing units (AMBU bags), sphygmomanometers and oxygen systems (cylinder, flowmeter, key).

The assessment of drugs and consumables revealed contrasting results – most commonly, supplies were either improved or deteriorated across all levels of facilities. The availability of oral and emergency contraceptive pills, intra-uterine contraceptive devices (IUCD-375), and most antibiotics (ampicillin, gentamycin, amoxicillin) increased across PHCs, CHC-level facilities and DHs, but so did the stock-out of condoms, pregnancy test kits, and the drug Amikacin. Improvement in the supply of uterotonics (Oxytocin, Misoprostol) was noted among PHC and CHC-level facilities, but not among DHs. On the other hand, the supply of antihypertensives (labetalol, nifedipine, methyldopa), drugs for the management of pre-eclampsia/ eclampsia (magnesium sulphate and calcium gluconate), iron and folic acid supplements, and oral rehydration solutions (ORS) mostly deteriorated among all categories of health facilities. Marked improvement was noted in the availability of Albendazole tablets (de-worming) and Vitamin A syrup (prevention of night blindness) across all levels of health facilities.

Table 1.2: Labor Room – physical condition and equipment

	PHC					CHC-level facilities					DH				
	CFA 2015 (n=405)		CFA 2016 (n=420)**		Change (% points)	CFA 2015 (n=95)		CFA 2016 (n=96)		Change (% points)	CFA 2015 (n=34)		CFA 2016 (n=34)		Change (% points)
	n	%	n	%		n	%	n	%		n	%	n	%	
Designated LR Available	**389**	96%	**414**	99%	3%	**94**	99%	**96**	100%	1%	**34**	100%	**34**	100%	0%
NBCC Available	352	87%	377	90%	3%	86	91%	91	95%	4%	31	91%	34	100%	9%
NBCC inside LR (among total NBCC available)	190	54%	253	67%	13%	47	55%	65	71%	17%	17	55%	30	88%	33%
In the facilities with designated LRs															
Cracks or seepage or plaster gets removed from LR wall on touch	196	50%	206	50%	-1%	38	40%	48	50%	10%	8	24%	13	38%	15%
Cracks or seepage or plaster gets removed from LR roof on touch	117	30%	150	36%	6%	25	27%	38	40%	13%	3	9%	10	29%	21%
LR with cracks or water seepage or plaster gets removed (wall or roof)	132	34%	187	45%	11%	25	27%	50	52%	25%	5	15%	15	44%	29%
LR floor with tiles/marbles or plastered	385	99%	408	99%	0%	92	98%	94	98%	0%	33	97%	33	97%	0%
LR in poor condition (any one problem in wall or roof or floor)	225	58%	233	56%	-2%	42	45%	55	57%	13%	10	29%	15	44%	15%
LR doesn't have inverter or generator: i.e. no power backup	2	1%	3	1%	0%	1	1%	0	0%	-1%	1	3%	0	0%	-3%

Continued

	PHC							CHC-level facilities							DH					
	CFA 2015 (n=405)		CFA 2016 (n=420)**		Change (% points)	CFA 2015 (n=95)		CFA 2016 (n=96)		Change (% points)	CFA 2015 (n=34)		CFA 2016 (n=34)		Change (% points)
	n	%	n	%		n	%	n	%		n	%	n	%	
Elbow tap absent in the handwashing station	240	62%	195	47%	-15%	47	50%	30	31%	-19%	9	26%	4	12%	-15%
Among all health facilities, stock-out or non-functional equipment in LR															
Radiant warmer (not available/ non-functional)	131	32%	109	26%	-6%	24	25%	15	16%	-10%	10	29%	3	9%	-21%
Cord Clamp	198	49%	122	29%	-20%	51	54%	27	28%	-26%	14	41%	6	18%	-24%
BP Apparatus (Digital/Mercury) any	210	52%	159	38%	-14%	36	38%	35	36%	-1%	12	35%	12	35%	0%
Mucus Extractor/sucker	202	50%	108	26%	-24%	45	47%	21	22%	-25%	8	24%	5	15%	-9%
Functional New Born weighing Machine (Digital)	306	76%	123	29%	-46%	63	66%	21	22%	-44%	22	65%	6	18%	-47%
Functional New Born weighing Machine (Manual)	94	23%	5	1%	-22%	18	19%	1	1%	-18%	6	18%	0	0%	-18%
AMBU Bag (250ml/500ml)	73	18%	14	3%	-15%	9	9%	3	3%	-6%	4	12%	1	3%	-9%
Neonatal Mask (O or 1 size)	188	46%	30	7%	-39%	40	42%	7	7%	-35%	11	32%	2	6%	-26%
Autoclave Machine	274	68%	58	14%	-54%	61	64%	8	8%	-56%	18	53%	2	6%	-47%
Oxygen cylinder, flowmeter and oxygen key	139	34%	127	30%	-4%	27	28%	20	21%	-8%	9	26%	3	9%	-18%

**PHC *Lakhisarai-Ramgarhchawk* did not have any data on equipment, drugs and consumables - hence denominator taken as (n=419) for calculating percentages under "stock-out or non-functional equipment"

Legends: CFA: comprehensive facility assessment; PHC: primary health center; CHC: community health center; DH: district hospital; LR: labor room; NBCC: newborn care corner; AMBU: artificial manual breathing unit

41

Table 1.3: Labor Room – stock-out of drugs and consumables

	PHC						CHC-level facilities						DH				
	CFA 2015 (n=405)		CFA 2016 (n=419)**		Change (% points)		CFA 2015 (n=95)		CFA 2016 (n=96)		Change (% points)		CFA 2015 (n=34)		CFA 2016 (n=34)		Change (% points)
	n	%	n	%			n	%	n	%			n	%	n	%	
Family planning																	
OCP (MALA-N or MALA-D)	144	36%	87	21%	-15%		35	37%	28	29%	-8%		15	44%	6	18%	-26%
ECPs	177	44%	83	20%	-24%		40	42%	20	21%	-21%		17	50%	12	35%	-15%
IUCD – 380A	77	19%	390	93%	74%		15	16%	92	96%	80%		7	21%	34	100%	79%
IUCD – 375	320	79%	141	34%	-45%		79	83%	30	31%	-52%		26	76%	7	21%	-56%
Condoms	148	37%	365	87%	51%		33	35%	79	82%	48%		16	47%	30	88%	41%
Pregnancy Test Kits (Nischay Kit)	209	52%	330	79%	27%		59	62%	71	74%	12%		17	50%	21	62%	12%
For management of labor (uterotonics, drugs for pre-eclampsia/ eclampsia)																	
Injection Oxytocin	123	30%	126	30%	0%		32	34%	24	25%	-9%		4	12%	4	12%	0%
Tablet Misoprostol	206	51%	179	43%	-8%		41	43%	33	34%	-9%		10	29%	10	29%	0%
Oxytocin and Misoprostol (both stock-out)	71	18%	78	19%	1%		18	19%	11	11%	-7%		2	6%	2	6%	0%
Any one uterotonic (Oxytocin/ Misoprostol) stock-out	258	64%	227	54%	-10%		55	58%	46	48%	-10%		12	35%	12	35%	0%
Injection Magnesium Sulphate	137	34%	174	42%	8%		27	28%	35	36%	8%		3	9%	6	18%	9%
Injection Calcium Gluconate	312	77%	327	78%	1%		70	74%	75	78%	4%		22	65%	22	65%	0%
Antihypertensives																	
Labetalol (injection or tablet)	402	99%	417	100%	0%		94	99%	96	100%	1%		31	91%	32	94%	3%

Continued

	PHC						CHC-level facilities						DH					
	CFA 2015 (n=405)		CFA 2016 (n=419)**		Change (% points)		CFA 2015 (n=95)		CFA 2016 (n=96)		Change (% points)		CFA 2015 (n=34)		CFA 2016 (n=34)		Change (% points)	
	n	%	n	%		n	%	n	%		n	%	n	%	
Capsule Nifedipine	341	84%	386	92%	8%	81	85%	89	93%	7%	26	76%	28	82%	6%
Tablet Methyl Dopa	389	96%	412	98%	2%	90	95%	94	98%	3%	33	97%	34	100%	3%
Injection Phytonadione (Vit. K1)	319	79%	319	76%	-3%	74	78%	77	80%	2%	21	62%	21	62%	0%
Antibiotics															
Capsule Ampicillin	358	88%	328	78%	-10%	88	93%	77	80%	-12%	28	82%	25	74%	-9%
Injection Gentamycin	191	47%	133	32%	-15%	37	39%	24	25%	-14%	13	38%	5	15%	-24%
Injection Amikacin	90	22%	194	46%	24%	17	18%	49	51%	33%	2	6%	12	35%	29%
Amoxicillin (injection or tablet)	193	48%	169	40%	-7%	52	55%	38	40%	-15%	14	41%	11	32%	-9%
Syrup Amoxicillin	348	86%	224	53%	-32%	76	80%	55	57%	-23%	25	74%	15	44%	-29%
For pregnant mother and children															
Syrup Iron Folic Acid with dispenser	172	42%	333	79%	37%	38	40%	74	77%	37%	15	44%	28	82%	38%
Tablet Iron Folic Acid – Large	120	30%	162	39%	9%	27	28%	29	30%	2%	12	35%	11	32%	-3%
Tablet Iron Folic Acid – Small	280	69%	289	69%	0%	69	73%	69	72%	-1%	26	76%	23	68%	-9%
Oral rehydration solutions (ORS)	10	2%	99	24%	21%	2	2%	24	25%	23%	4	12%	9	26%	15%
Syrup Salbutamol	376	93%	345	82%	-11%	91	96%	75	78%	-18%	28	82%	28	82%	0%
Tablet Salbutamol	91	22%	no data			24	25%	no data			9	26%	no data		
Tablet Albendazole	81	20%	26	6%	-14%	22	23%	20	21%	-2%	12	35%	3	9%	-26%
Syrup Albendazole	160	40%	224	53%	14%	43	45%	55	57%	12%	12	35%	15	44%	9%
Tablet Dicyclomine	145	36%	no data			32	34%	no data			13	38%	no data		

Continued

	PHC					CHC-level facilities					DH				
	CFA 2015 (n=405)		CFA 2016 (n=419)**		Change (% points)	CFA 2015 (n=95)		CFA 2016 (n=96)		Change (% points)	CFA 2015 (n=34)		CFA 2016 (n=34)		Change (% points)
	n	%	n	%		n	%	n	%		n	%	n	%	
Zinc Sulphate dispersible tablet 10mg	391	97%	409	98%	1%	89	94%	95	99%	5%	31	91%	33	97%	6%
Zinc Sulphate dispersible tablet 20mg	134	33%	224	53%	20%	43	45%	50	52%	7%	18	53%	23	68%	15%
Syrup Vitamin-A	285	70%	222	53%	-17%	77	81%	54	56%	-25%	29	85%	14	41%	-44%

**PHC *Lakhisarai-Ramgarhchawk* did not have any data on equipment, drugs and consumables.

Legends: CFA: comprehensive facility assessment; PHC: primary health center; CHC: community health center; DH: district hospital;OCP: oral contraceptive pill; ECP: emergency contraceptive pill; IUCD: intrauterine contraceptive device

1.3.2.2 Availability of human resources

Table 1.4 depicts data on the availability of human resources, in terms of the proportion of each

level of health facility that recorded presence of an adequate number (as defined earlier in the

Methods section) of healthcare providers by cadre.

At the PHC level, 99% of facilities reported having adequate medical officers (primary care

physicians) and 91% reported having adequate staff nurses during CFA 2015 – and this further

increased 1 percentage-point in 2016. While 93% of the CHC-level facilities reported presence

of adequate medical officers during either assessment, only 44% of DHs did so in 2016 – a 6

percentage-points reduction from the 2015 status. The availability of staff nurses increased 28

percentage-points among CHC-level facilities, and increased 24 percentage-points across DHs –

yet only 45% CHC-level facilities and 26% DHs reported having an adequate number of nurses

available for service in 2016. Similarly, while the number of specialist physicians increased

between 5% and 20 percentage-points at both CHC-level facilities and DHs between 2015 and

2016, 75% facilities in either category still lacked the adequate number of anaesthesiologists or

pediatricians, and 60% lacked general surgeons. Adequate number of OBGYNs were present

only in 31% CHC-level facilities and in 47% DHs during CFA 2016.

Table 1.4: Facilities with adequate personnel

	PHC					CHC-level facilities					DH				
	CFA 2015** (n=404)		CFA 2016 (n=420)		Change (% points)	CFA 2015** (n=94)		CFA 2016 (n=96)		Change (% points)	CFA 2015 (n=34)		CFA 2016 (n=34)		Change (% points)
	n	%	n	%		n	%	n	%		n	%	n	%	
Medical Officers (primary care providers)	400	99%	420	100%	1%	87	93%	89	93%	0%	17	50%	15	44%	-6%
Nursing staff (ANM & GNM)	368	91%	386	92%	1%	16	17%	43	45%	28%	1	3%	9	26%	24%
Obstetrician & Gynecologists (OBGYN)						19	20%	30	31%	11%	11	32%	16	47%	15%
Pediatricians			not applicable			19	20%	24	25%	5%	5	15%	8	24%	9%
General Surgeons						17	18%	37	39%	20%	11	32%	14	41%	9%
Anesthesiologists						15	16%	24	25%	9%	4	12%	8	24%	12%

**Human resources data not available from 1 PHC and 1 CHC during CFA 2015

Legends: CFA: comprehensive facility assessment; PHC: primary health center; CHC: community health center; DH: district hospital;ANM: auxiliary nurse midwives; GNM: general nurse midwives

1.4 Discussion

In Bihar, as the government and its development partners recognized the need to address system-level deficiencies, they clearly envisioned that strengthening the foundational components of the public health system would be the correct starting point. At the same time, they also made a conscious decision to do so through keeping the focus on strategies that would most likely improve RMNCH. Therefore, the BTSP can be best described as an example of a program adopting the diagonal approach to HSS[74] – one that starts with a focus on specific programmatic outcomes but strives to achieve these through identifying and addressing bottlenecks across the health system. Such an approach is often preferred to ensure maximum utilization of existing health system resources through synchronizing vertical health programs and horizontal systemic interventions, and works particularly well in addressing health conditions that require a continuum-of-care approach, like RMNCH and chronic diseases. Further, when supported by purposeful health governance and efficient financing, the gains in disease control programs and primary care achieved through the diagonal approach can potentially be sustained, even in absence of external support.[75]

The current paper presents the genesis of Bihar's HSS program. As the state transitioned to a new governance era in 2005, there was an initial government-level focus on improving the most urgent and sensitive health parameters like immunization coverage, institutional deliveries, and health workforce vacancies (especially FLWs). A 2007 Government of India task force report on Bihar's health sector had recommended strengthening the public health infrastructure, developing a skilled workforce, and ensuring the supply of essential drugs and equipment as key to achieving sustainable reductions in maternal and infant mortality rates, fertility rate and malnutrition. Home-based maternal and newborn care provision, ensuring skilled birth attendance and facility-based emergency obstetric care services, integrated management of neonatal and childhood diseases, increasing breastfeeding practices and immunization coverage, behavior change communication, and better nutritional provision through ICDS were identified as the key strategies to achieve these goals.[76] The IFHI was a welcome first step in this direction, wherein the government collaborated with external funders and development partners to expand facility-based and outreach-based service coverage to pregnant women, mothers and children. There was a simultaneous push to improve the quality of care through training of nursing staff and enabling the FLWs to better manage client needs through using mobile technology. Definitive progress was also noted towards developing systems for collecting, managing, and analyzing facility-level data to understand and address the system gaps.

The experiences gained during the IFHI phase were instrumental in motivating the government and its partners to expand the scope of the ongoing vertical programs, and indeed look at opportunities to address the system-level barriers while still working towards the same outcomes (the diagonal approach). Through these years (2011-2013) of collaborative work, the development partners felt confident that the state government had the political will and intent to invest in long-term goals of strengthening Bihar's public health system.[44] These factors supported the launch of BTSP in November 2013 as a state-wide HSS effort that would work to strengthen the state health apparatus. The current paper not only describes the novel health governance mechanism put in place to implement the expansive HSS program, but also highlights some of the specific processes through which BTSP envisioned to improve the foundational elements of Bihar's public health system. The following sections deliberate on three key issues emerging from the paper – the necessity to focus on the foundational elements of

Bihar's public health system, the BTSP's targeted approach to address human resources

shortcomings, and the persistent challenges within Bihar's supply chain system.

1.4.1 Justifying the HSS approach

The 2007 WHO HSS framework identifies six inter-related and dynamically interacting

"building blocks" which represent the six core functions of a health system: service delivery,

human resources, medical products, vaccines, and technologies (i.e. supplies and logistics),

health information systems, health financing, and governance. The framework emphasizes that

siloed actions within individual building blocks will never translate into HSS, but multi-sectorial

interventions are required to bring about meaningful changes in access to, and coverage of

locally essential services, while improving the quality and safety of care delivery.[77] While

focusing on increasing public health financing and making it efficient remains a cornerstone of

expanding services and covering more people, understanding and addressing gaps at the facility-

level through supply-side investments has been emphasized as an equally important step in HSS.

Analysis of district-level household survey data for the 8 EAG states in India revealed that while

presence of a PHC greater than 10 kms away from one's residence decreased the likelihood of

institutional deliveries by over 50%, presence of adequate infrastructure, essential equipment and

laboratory services, along with physicians and skilled nurses significantly increased the

utilization of services.[78] A recent systematic review on health system challenges in providing

quality midwifery services in India found that both poorer states like Odisha as well as those

better-off like Maharashtra suffered from acute shortage of skilled nurses. In many of these

settings, absence of proper infrastructure and essential supplies at all levels of the public health

facilities had significant negative impact on nurses' job performance and motivation.[79]

Investing in infrastructure and logistics has been recognized in the WHO HSS framework as a basic and necessary requirement for satisfactory health service delivery, and it requires a complex process of financing and purchase-related decision-making. Simultaneously, the importance of efficient distribution of the existing health workforce, while supporting policies to improve their performance, had also been emphasized upon.[77]As part of a multi-country investment case study to examine health system needs for an equitable scale-up of RMNCH services, researchers focused on two districts in Odisha – which, like Bihar, is one of the poorer, predominantly rural, EAG states in India. The case study overwhelmingly revealed a critical necessity to address gaps in basic facility-level infrastructure, human resources, and essential supplies – like the need to re-design/ construct nearly one-third of the sub-centers; equip PHCs to enable them deliver BEmONC services; establish blood banks at CHCs to achieve CEmONC service capability; manage stock-ins of essential drugs and supplies; and planning to redistribute the workforce as per needs while creating opportunities for training and further capacity building. The research team found that only one-fifth of all public health facilities in either district satisfied the Indian Public Health Standards in terms of infrastructure and human resource needs.[80]

These findings from the EAG states, especially Odisha, closely resemble the status of the public health system in Bihar at the end of 2013, and clearly substantiate the BTSP's approach in targeting facility-level improvements in infrastructure, human resources and essential supplies as fundamental necessities for delivering strengthened RMNCH services.

1.4.2 Prioritizing limited human resources

The BTSP provided technical assistance to the state government to rationalize the process of human resource management through prioritizing the most urgent needs at different levels of health facilities. For example, the process aimed to ensure at least 1 medical officer and 3

nursing staff at each PHC for BEmONC service provision, while also striving to meet the more

demanding requirements at CHC-level facilities and DHs which were mandated to provide

CEmONC services (details in the Methods section). The most fruitful reflection of this policy

was at the PHC-level: all facilities reported having at least 1 medical officer on duty, while 92%

had an adequate number of nursing staff by 2016. For the CHC-level facilities, while 93% had an

adequate number of medical officers (at least 2 per facility), only 45% met the criteria for having

the minimum number (at least 10) of nurses. The problem was more severe at the DHs with only

44% having an adequate number (at least 11) of medical officers. Only 26% of DHs had

adequate (at least 45) nursing staff. With regards to the specialist physician positions, between

50% to 75% of the CHC-level facilities and DHs lacked the minimum number (at least 1 each for

CHCs and 2 each for DHs) of OBGYNs, anaesthesiologists, pediatricians or surgeons.

Non-availability of specialist physicians at CHC-level facilities had been reported from Uttar

Pradesh, an EAG state like Bihar. Based on the 2012-13 District-Level Household Survey, over

60% of CHCs in the state functioned without any specialist physicians, and typically remote

facilities had the least availability. The shortfall of anesthesiologists, surgeons and pediatricians

was over 80% of the total need as per the Indian Public Health Standards, while that for

OBGYNs was over 70%.[81] Availability of specialist physicians in the public health system had

been a long-standing problem in even socio-economically better-off states like Andhra Pradesh

and Telangana, where researchers found 1 pediatrician for every 10 neonatal intensive care unit

beds (instead of the recommended 1:4 ratio) across public secondary and tertiary health facilities

– and this was linked to the delivery of poor quality of care.[82] An analysis of the National

Sample Survey data revealed that as of January 2016, Bihar had only 5 physicians, nurses and midwives per 10,000 population – the lowest among all states – while the national average was 21/10,000 population. The concentration of doctors in the state was 3.3 per 10,000 population against a national average of 11.3, while that of nurses & midwives was 2 against a national average of 9.4.[83]

The staffing pattern exhibited during the initial years of the BTSP presents a picture of prioritization on one hand, and of the continuing severe shortage of trained human resources on the other. Clearly, the BTSP had put an onus on ensuring that the PHCs remained functional as the first point of institutional care that could provide BEmONC services – an approach that was efficient because these facilities catered to the primary health care needs of the population. While staffing requirements were more challenging to meet at the higher-level facilities (especially for specialist physicians), it is understandable that creating additional trained workforce requires time and investments in nursing and medical schools – and this can certainly be considered as a major unfinished task. Inadequate numbers of medical officers and nursing staff, although extremely undesirable, do not wholly compromise the functionality of CHC-level facilities or DHs. However, the dismal availability of specialist physicians is bound to impact the ability to provide CEmONC services. In reality, most PHCs and CHC-level facilities in Bihar struggle to meet all BEmONC signal functions[38],while blood banks are not consistently present at all DHs which deliver CEmONC services. Unless these limitations are addressed with urgency, the situation could adversely impact efforts to reduce maternal and childhood morbidity and mortality in the state.

1.4.3 The challenges within Bihar's supply chain system

The analysis of CFA 2015 and 2016 data revealed contrasting pictures of Bihar's supply chain system. On one hand, the availability of essential equipment like functional autoclaves, oxygen cylinders, radiant warmers, mucous extractors, baby weighing machines, and AMBU bags with neonatal oxygen masks improved across all types of health facilities. However, data on the availability of drugs and consumables showed that while certain supplies like contraceptive pills, antibiotics, Vitamin A syrup uniformly increased across PHCs, CHC-level facilities and DHs, the supply of antihypertensives, iron and folic acid supplements and ORS was majorly affected. An assessment of 85 PHC and CHC-level facilities in terms of the capacity to provide hypertension and diabetes-related care across 24 districts in Madhya Pradesh (an EAG state, like Bihar) revealed a comparable picture.[84]Less than 50% of the surveyed PHCs had glucometers or weighing machines, and less than one-third of CHCs had functional ECG machines. The availability of standard antihypertensives varied widely. While 84% PHCs had stocks of calcium channel blockers and 68% had beta blockers, over 90% of CHCs reported availability of these two drugs. In contrast, diuretics were available in less than one-third of CHCs and in less than one-fifth of the PHCs. Among the anti-diabetic medicines, only metformin was available at over two-thirds PHCs or CHCs, while insulin was in short supply at nearly 60% CHCs and 90% PHCs. Low dose aspirin was available at only 50% CHCs and 44% PHCs.

Such mixed results clearly signal ongoing challenges within a state's supply chain including supply-side budgeting, procurement and/or distribution. While an established Bihar Medical Services & Infrastructure Corporation Limited exists to manage the physical infrastructure and supplies needs of Bihar, the process also depends on local-level mechanisms. These include, empanelling approved vendors to directly manage inventory at the facility level, as well as the capacity of the district-level health officials to utilize the Logistics Management Information System to prevent stock-outs. Finally, all of these processes are critically dependent on the state's health financing system – in terms of both the allocation of funds and their utilization.Berman et al.[24] had noted that public health spending in Bihar was not only insufficient but also inefficient, since only 69%-79% of the total budgetary allocation in health was actually utilized between 2007-08 and 2013-14. Notably over this period, spending on primary care as a proportion of total government health expenditure (TGHE) remained stable between 65%-74%, mainly due to federal financing support through the NRHM (almost 45% of TGHE in 2013-14). However, real per capita expenditure (in 2004-05 INR) on primary care increased modestly: from INR 92 (USD 1.3) in 2007-08 to INR 112 (USD 1.6) in 2013-14, signaling a lack of meaningful increase in state-level funding. It was concluded that Bihar's public health system clearly lacked the capacity to develop an outcome-based financing system, resulting in wastage and redundancy. It was emphasized that organizational changes needed to be implemented to make best use of the limited resources – through developing electronic financial management systems, operational research capacity within the health department to ensure close monitoring of outcomes and evidence-based decision-making, and increasing system-wide transparency and accountability.

1.4.4 Limitations

The current paper relied on the analysis of existing programmatic data that was generated through the 2015 and 2016 CFAs. During these initial years of the BTSP, the CFAs were restricted to collecting data on human resource availability and the condition of the labor rooms in terms of infrastructure and supplies. Hence, the analysis was accordingly bound by the limited information available from this data. From 2017 onward, the CFAs were expanded to include more facility-level parameters, and the authors shall look to analyze this progress in the future. As such, any analysis based on limited programmatic data will continue to have similar limitations.

Further, from a programmatic aspect, the one major drawback of the CFA-based planning of inputs might be the reliance on cross-sectional assessments and not on the status across the year. This is particularly the case for medical supplies and equipment, whose stock-out/ functionality status may change overnight, or the availability of certain drugs may depend on seasonal demands – such as Vitamin A syrup during the half-yearly campaigns. Obviously, cross-sectional assessments may not always reflect the true functional status of a facility. However, as pointed out earlier, these shortcomings can be addressed through better and more efficient use of the Logistics Management Information System, and need not depend on the data from the CFAs.

1.5 Conclusion

Given this evidence, the current paper finds that BTSP has progressively strengthened the health system although concerning issues remain. Recollecting the fact that as of 2014-15, there were only 60% functional PHCs and 9% functional CHCs in Bihar along with 75% vacancies in physician positions[21, 24], it is understandable that it shall take much more time, effort and investment to address the shortcomings in infrastructure, essential supplies and human resources in the public health facilities. In this regard, the HSS approach adopted by the BTSP seems to be justified and well-rooted in evidence. Further, the current analysis also highlights the importance of the CFAs as key for ground-level needs assessment and bottom-up planning for HSS, and strongly endorses the continuation of such exhaustive periodic exercises.

The two critical areas that should warrant urgent attention from the BTSP include the staffing status at the facilities above the PHC level, and addressing supply chain issues at the local levels. While the shortage of specialist physicians is a common problem across state health systems in India and more globally, the absence of an adequate number of nursing staff at the CHC-level facilities and DHs is perhaps more worrying and is likely an issue that can be addressed even within the limitations of Bihar's health system. Similarly, while increasing and reforming health financing in Bihar may be a lengthy process, future CFAs (or other focused operational research studies) can surely look to identify local issues that adversely impact the supply chain system. In this regard, training the facility-level and district-level health officials to use the Logistics Management Information System more efficiently can perhaps address some of these problems. This paper recommends that the BTSP urgently look to focus on these areas as part of its techno-managerial support to the Bihar government.

Finally, it remains important to appreciate that the evolution of BTSP represents a critical transformation of the collaborative approach between the Bihar government and its development partners. While the partner agencies were driving an intensive ground-level implementation process during the IFHI phase, their roles gradually changed to providing techno-managerial and capacity building support to the state-wide public health system during the BTSP phase. The interventions were co-designed with the government functionaries who were made active partners in generating data and understanding the evidence, and were further encouraged to track progress through the joint review forums. These steps were designed to put emphasis on accountability, as well as to ensure a steady and smooth transfer of ownership. Some good examples include the gradual evolution of the nurse-mentoring program, and the integration of the SRU and DRUs (which started with co-positioning of BTSP staff) into the state health apparatus. Learnings from BTSP are also being implemented in other states of India through contextual customization – for example, the technological innovations for FLWs have been scaled up as job tools.[54]

While the BTSP was initially funded for a four-year period (2014-2017), the support is being currently sustained to ensure the continuity of this process. The overall findings from this paper should encourage the state health policymakers, who are active stakeholders in the BTSP, to continue their support for the facility-level interventions and necessarily become more engaged partners with a vision towards long-term sustainability. Indeed, this diagonal HSS program is a promising endeavor to gradually progress towards a more efficient, sustainable and equitable public health system in Bihar.

Chapter 2: Measuring the structural readiness of public health facilities: findings from the 2017 and 2019 comprehensive facility assessments in Bihar, India

2.1 Introduction

The public health system in Bihar – a predominantly-rural, densely populated, and socio-economically disadvantaged state in eastern India with 104 million population (2011 census) – had long suffered from systemic underfunding and the lack of planned investments in developing its infrastructure, supply chain (including provision of basic medicines and equipment) and skilled health workforce.[11, 24, 25] Compared to its population-based needs, Bihar in 2014 recorded a 40% shortage in the number of functional primary health centers and 90% shortage in the number of functional community health centers (first referral level). Consequently, nearly 80% of the population were compelled to seek necessary care from the formal and informal private sector, incurring significant out-of-pocket expenses.[21, 24, 26]

Recognizing this, in November 2013, the state embarked on a diagonal approach to strengthen its public health system – one that starts with a focus on specific programmatic outcomes, but strives to achieve these through identifying and addressing bottlenecks across the health system. This initiative – the Bihar Technical Support Program (BTSP) – was funded by the Gates Foundation with CARE India as the lead implementation partner and evolved through previous years of collaborative facility-based and outreach-based programs. Though the program focused on improvement across reproductive, maternal, newborn and child health (RMNCH) and nutrition outcomes, the development partners also provided technical assistance to the Bihar government to identify and address structural gaps in the state's public health system. Details on the genesis of the BTSP, its integration within the state health system, and the innovative health governance mechanism had been discussed in the first paper of this book.

Since its inception in November 2013, the BTSP had closely aligned itself with India's national reproductive, maternal, newborn, child and adolescent health (RMNCH+A) program which was launched earlier that year. The national RMNCH+A strategy involved a continuum-of-care approach to address the health and nutritional needs of a female child across her life-cycle: infancy (newborn), childhood, adolescence, reproductive age and maternity. The program envisioned purposeful collaborations between the federal/state government and development partners to address the systemic shortcomings in infrastructure, human resources, supply chain and referral services at the local levels through data-driven program monitoring and supervision – thereby prioritizing health system strengthening as a key means to achieve program goals.[59, 60] Under the RMNCH+A program, the federal government identified 184 underperforming districts across the country (termed as "high priority districts") by selecting 25% of the under-performing districts within each state based on performance parameters.[85] Bihar had 10 high priority districts identified under this federal scheme – *Jamui, Saharsa, Purnia, Sitamarhi, Sheohar, East Champaran, Araria, Katihar, Kishanganj*, and *Gaya*.[86] The national program emphasized the need to identify all health facilities within a state that conducted deliveries ("delivery points"), and focus on strengthening these sites to deliver comprehensive RMNCH+A services. The program proposed a one-year time frame to renovate existing facilities where required, and a two-year timeline to construct new primary and community health centers (or similar facilities), with concomitant emphasis on ensuring transport services for efficient referral of emergency cases. The program recognized that skilled human resources shortage existed across all levels of the public health care delivery system, but stressed that states must prioritize the lowest level of facilities conducting deliveries (as these were closest to the communities), more so in their most disadvantaged districts. It was further suggested to develop plans for decentralized human resources recruitment at the district level, while rationalizing the process to maximize service coverage, prioritizing the rural and remote areas. The long-term goal remained to develop basic emergency obstetric and newborn care (BEmONC) service capability at all primary health centers, and comprehensive emergency obstetric and newborn care (CEmONC) service capability at all higher-level facilities.[60, 85]

While the BTSP embraced most of the priority areas outlined under the national program, it also recognized that given the realities of Bihar's public health system, it was necessary to start with addressing three "foundational elements"[29] – infrastructure, supply chain and workforce. In this regard, the priority was to identify existing gaps, collecting data to assess the current state of affairs and subsequently monitor project progress. To serve this need, CARE India instituted a structurally embedded but functionally independent Concurrent Measurement and Learning unit which conducted comprehensive assessments of all public health facilities in the state that conducted deliveries – known as comprehensive facility assessments (CFAs). The initial CFAs conducted in 2015 and 2016 involved a limited assessment of human resources and labor room infrastructure and supplies, but the subsequent assessments conducted in 2017 and 2019 expanded to not only include more details on workforce, infrastructure and supplies, but also to cover other areas like maternity wards, laboratories, drug storage rooms, and referral transport systems. The progress and challenges in structural improvement of Bihar's public health facilities as evidenced through CFA 2015 and 2016 have been described in details in the first paper of this book.

The current (second) paper continues the quantitative assessment of facility readiness (structural readiness), utilizing comprehensive data generated by CARE India through the expanded CFAs conducted in 2017 and 2019. Specifically, the objectives of the current study were to: (1) conduct a comparative assessment of the status of facility readiness in the public health facilities of Bihar between 2017 (at end of the first four years of BTSP) and 2019, and describe the continuation of progress or lack thereof; (2) quantify the facility readiness through a scoring system that would reflect the core facility-level interventions under BTSP; and (3) compare the change in this score over time (2015, 2017 and 2019) across different districts and levels of health facilities in Bihar. "Facility readiness" was operationalized in terms of the availability of a number of facility-level characteristics such as infrastructure, human resources, stock-in of functional equipment, consumables and drugs, referral transport systems, laboratory services, infection control and biomedical waste management practices. The first objective was addressed by analyzing data generated through the 2017 and 2019 CFAs conducted by CARE India's Concurrent Measurement and Learning unit. The next two objectives were addressed by developing a "facility-level maternal and newborn care (MNC) structural readiness score" – henceforth referred to as facility readiness score, based on a common set of indicators from CFA 2015, 2017 and 2019, and using this score to map the change at 2-year intervals, from 2015 to 2019.

2.2 Methods

2.2.1 The CFA methodology

The CFAs were executed as annual/ biennial cross-sectional assessments of all "functional" public health facilities in Bihar, defined as facilities which conducted at least 100 deliveries in the year preceding the CFA (*also referred to as delivery points, keeping in-sync with the terminology used by the national RMNCH+A program*). For the state of Bihar, such delivery points included Level 2 (primary health centers, community health centers and referral hospitals) and Level 3 (sub-divisional hospitals and district hospitals) health facilities. This categorization (as per Levels) reflects the hierarchy followed by the state health system, and doesn't exactly correspond to BEmONC or CEmONC service delivery capacity. It is worth noting that ideally, all Level 2 facilities in Bihar are expected to provide at least BEmONC services, while all Level 3 facilities are expected to provide CEmONC services. However, in reality, not all Level 2 facilities in Bihar can perform the 7 WHO BEmONC signal functions.[38] On the other hand, among the Level 3 facilities, some sub-divisional hospitals can only provide BEmONC services while blood banks (a key CEmONC signal function) are not present in most facilities. The current study follows the Level 2/ Level 3 categorization. The village-level health sub-centers (Level 1 facilities) rarely conduct deliveries and therefore were not included in the CFAs; while Medical Colleges (Level 3 multi-specialty centers) remained outside the scope of BTSP's work. Four CFAs have been conducted to date – in 2015, 2016, 2017 and 2019. Each CFA represented a census of delivery points in each of the 38 districts of Bihar during the respective periods of assessment (i.e., no sampling was done). The methodology and results of the 2015 and 2016 CFAs have been described in the first paper of this book.

The 2017 CFA was conducted between September and December 2017 and covered 550 functional delivery points, while the 2019 CFA was conducted in August-September 2019 and covered 552 functional delivery points. To implement the CFAs, the Concurrent Measurement and Learning unit developed a standardized questionnaire guided by the National Quality Assurance Standards guidelines and tools, and the Maternal and Newborn Health toolkit.[39, 40] During the first two CFAs (2015 and 2016), data was collected on the availability of human

resources and condition of the labor rooms (including infrastructure and essential supplies).
However, the scope of data collection was expanded during the 2017 and 2019 CFAs to include
information on maternity wards, referral transport services, bio-medical waste management and
infection control, laboratory services, operating rooms and drug storage facilities, as well as
other useful information.

Data collection for the CFAs was conducted by trained staff employed/ hired by the BTSP. Prior
to each CFA, rigorous refresher training was conducted for about 10 days, specifically focussing
on the dedicated tools. This was considered necessary in view of the expanded nature of the 2017
and 2019 CFAs, and between 4 to 8 days were required per facility for completion of the data
collection exercise. The data collection in 2017 and 2019 was done through hand-held android
tablets (tablet-sized personal computer devices) using a hybrid custom-built platform enabled
with inherent logic checks developed in-house, bridging between the proprietary licensed
Survey-CTO platform [87] and the Open Data Kit (free and open-source software) platform [88]. The
data collection teams conducted direct observation of infrastructure (e.g., condition of wall,
floor, roof, amenities etc.), checked the functionality of available equipment, physically counted
available drugs and consumables, and observed the measures in-place for infection control, biomedical waste management and disposal of condemned (junk) articles. They collected data on
availability of functional (on-road) ambulances and their service delivery in the 30 days prior to
the CFA (cross-checked with register logs), the types and number of laboratory tests performed
in the last 30 days before the CFA, and the use of web-based software (*e-Aushadhi*) in the
facility drug storage room. The teams further collected detailed data on availability of the
different health workforce cadres in each facility, noting the number of staff who had been
recruited under the regular recruitment process, those hired as contractual employees (i.e. hired

under different projects as term-limited employees), the staff that were deputed-in (transferred in for a limited time period) from another facility, as well as any employee who was currently deputed-out (transferred out for a limited time period) to another facility or was absent from service for at least 3 months.

To ensure the quality of the data being collected (in addition to the built-in logic checks described above), the district measurement, learning and evaluation (MLE) officers, data quality monitoring coordinators, and external monitors (Oxford Policy Management during CFA 2019) conducted random spot-checks in almost 50% of the assessed facilities.

2.2.2 Data analysis

2.2.2.1 The descriptive analysis

The data generated through the 2017 and 2019 CFAs (available with the Concurrent Measurement and Learning unit of CARE India) was analyzed using STATA SE v.15.[41] Since a vast amount of data was collected from different departments of a facility like labor rooms, maternity wards, and laboratories, the descriptive analysis was organized under distinct domains (described below) to facilitate a better understanding of the health system strengthening approach. This data was presented as the number (percentage) of Level 2 and Level 3 facilities that satisfied each assessment parameter during CFA 2017 vs. CFA 2019, for the domains of – infrastructure; stock-in of equipment, consumables and drugs – defined as the availability of at least one functional equipment/ any stock-in quantity of a consumable or a drug on the day of visit; infection control and biomedical waste management practices; referral transport system (ambulance availability and service delivery in last 30 days); laboratory services (tests conducted in last 30 days); and management of drug stores (use of the web-based software, *e-Aushadhi*).

For the human resources domain, the data was analyzed and presented as the number of positions sanctioned, the number and percentage of positions filled (against sanctioned positions), and the change in percentage availability between the two CFAs. The number of staff available for service was calculated as [number of staff (posted through regular recruitment + deputed-in) - number of staff (deputed-out + absent for 3 months or more)]. This calculation excluded all contractual employees who had been hired under various ongoing state and national health programs, but those numbers have been presented in text. The analysis was done separately for Level 2 and Level 3 health facilities, and for each cadre of health care worker, including general duty medical officers (primary care physicians), specialist doctors (internal medicine physicians, obstetricians & gynecologists or OBGYNs, anesthesiologists, pediatricians and general surgeons), nursing staff (general nurse midwives (GNM) and auxiliary nurse midwives (ANM)). Data on additional staff positions collected only during CFA 2019 was also analyzed.

It is worthwhile to note that the current analysis of human resource data differed from the approach adopted during data analysis for CFA 2015 and 2016. Previously, the focus had been on assessing the "adequacy" of each cadre of the health workforce at each type of facility, as per the 2012 revised Indian Public Health Standards.[42] For example, the availability of 1 general duty medical officer at a primary health center or at least 11 medical officers at a district hospital was considered to be "adequate" presence of this cadre for the specific type of health facility. However, during CFA 2017 and 2019 it was decided to impose a higher standard by calculating the proportion of the total number of government-sanctioned positions (for each facility, for each cadre) in which the personnel were actually available for service. The number of sanctioned positions for any cadre at any health facility was usually higher than the number required for adequacy, and this was particularly true for Level 2 facilities. It was hoped that this approach might motivate policymakers to sanction focussed recruitment drives targeting the vacancies which critically compromised service delivery, while also allowing flexibility in changing the sanctioned numbers for different cadres to realistically meet the recruitment goals (like more nursing staff at primary health centers instead of specialists).

2.2.2.2 Development of the facility readiness score

While the detailed data on structural aspects of each functional delivery point in Bihar was extremely useful for assessing the ongoing development process and planning around areas that needed attention, it was not particularly helpful to facilitate a quick understanding of progress at policymaking levels. Ever since the first CFA was conducted, there had been ongoing deliberations within the BTSP leadership (government and partner organizations) to develop an operational scoring system for Bihar's public health facilities that could also be used to provide feedback to the national RMNCH+A program.

Initially, it was thought that including each assessment parameter in the CFAs to formulate a simple facility readiness score, where equal weightage would be accorded to all items to avoid any bias was adequate. Since the data was analyzed as binary responses (yes or no) to the presence or absence of a specific parameter, all negatively framed responses could easily be reverse-coded, so that a higher score would reflect better facility readiness. While such a scoring system was feasible with the limited data collected during 2015 and 2016 CFAs, it posed challenges with the expanded data collection in 2017 and 2019 CFAs. First, including hundreds of items to construct this score, though technically possible, was viewed as inefficient and impractical. Second, since data was now being collected on almost all structural aspects of a public health facility, the data represented elements that were currently beyond the scope of BTSP's RMNCH-centric system strengthening interventions. That is, while all improvements within a public health facility would be extremely desirable findings, not all can be directly attributed to BTSP's core work. Further, such a score would certainly not be useful to be reported to the national RMNCH+A program.

To overcome this challenge, it seemed prudent to focus on selecting a limited number of parameters that would reflect the changes in human resources, infrastructure and essential supplies related to delivering maternal and newborn care services at the health facilities. In other words, it was proposed to develop a score that would reflect the facility-level structural readiness for MNC (maternal and newborn care). There were two key reasons behind this choice. First, many of the interventions to improve reproductive health, child health and nutritional status of pregnant women and children were typically outreach-based activities with limited role for the clinics. For example, reproductive health services involved delivering behavior change communication regarding family planning methods, their benefits towards health, related decision-making and availability of services by the frontline health workers. Similarly, nutritional and child health-related interventions were mostly delivered at the community level by *Anganwadi* workers under the Integrated Child Development Services (ICDS) program. . The health facilities had limited roles in these areas, like conducting family planning counseling clinics, fixed-day services, and maintaining supplies of contraceptives, vitamin A syrups, iron and folic acid tablets and deworming tablets. Second, a set of basic MNC-centric parameters would be relevant for all levels of health facilities (ranging from primary health centers to district hospitals), and would be common across all the CFAs. In other words, such a score would allow the assessment of progress for all facilities across the different CFAs.

Based on these considerations, through an iterative process of consultation between the implementation team (policymakers at the state level along with a select group of district and block-level health care providers) and the technical support team (CARE India leadership ground team, and public health experts), a list of 44 indicators were selected. As depicted in **Panel 2.1**, these indicators addressed the human resources, infrastructure and essential supplies (equipment, consumables, medicines) domains, and were reflective of the service-specific structural readiness for management of normal deliveries and emergency management of postpartum hemorrhage, newborn care (including management of asphyxia) and infection prevention. In selecting these 44 parameters, the group also considered the list of minimum essential commodities proposed under the Government of India's RMNCH+A program.[89]

In order to calculate the facility readiness score, each parameter in Panel 2.1 was awarded a score of 1 for its presence and 0 for absence (opposite scoring for negatively-framed questions) – so that a higher score represented better structural readiness. If data was not collected for a particular parameter at a facility, it was awarded 0 points. Thus, the possible score range for each facility was 0-44. The actual score for each facility was next transformed to a 0-10 scale using the formula: $transformed\ (final)\ score = \left(\left(\frac{10-0}{44-0}\right) * (X - 44)\right) + 10$, where X is the original facility readiness score.

Panel 2.1: Indicators used to develop Facility Readiness Score

Sl. No.	Indicators	Domains	Management of normal deliveries and emergency management of PPH	Newborn care (including management of asphyxia)	Infection prevention
			Service-specific readiness		
1	At least one ANM or GNM Nurse available for service	Human Resources	x	x	x
2	At least one Pediatrician available for service	Human Resources		x	x
3	At least one OBGYN available for service	Human Resources	x	x	x
4	At least one General Duty Medical Officer/ Internal Medicine Physician available for service	Human Resources	x	x	x
5	All walls in LR have at least 6 feet tiles	Infrastructure	x	x	x
6	No sign of water seepage from wall or roof in LR	Infrastructure	x	x	x
7	Facility has a new born care corner inside the LR	Infrastructure		x	
8	No area with diameter 1 feet or more in the LR roof where plaster is chipped-off	Infrastructure	x	x	x
9	At least 1 invertor/generator (power back-up) available in LR	Infrastructure	x	x	
10	Elbow tap available in LR	Infrastructure	x	x	x
	Availability of at least one functional:	Supplies - Equipment			
11	digital/manual baby weighing machine in LR	Supplies - Equipment		x	
12	radiant warmer in LR	Supplies - Equipment		x	
13	BP apparatus (digital/mercury) in Facility	Supplies - Equipment	x		
14	stethoscope in Facility	Supplies - Equipment	x		
15	Fetal Doppler/Fetoscope in Facility	Supplies - Equipment	x	x	
16	Haemoglobinometer in Facility	Supplies - Equipment	x		
17	Pulse oximeter in Facility	Supplies - Equipment	x		

Continued

Sl. No.	Indicators	Domains	Service-specific readiness		
			Management of normal deliveries and emergency management of PPH	Newborn care (including management of asphyxia)	Infection prevention
18	Phototherapy machine in LR			x	
19	Suction machine (Electric / Foot Operated) in LR			x	
20	AMBU Bag (250 ml or 500 ml) in LR			x	
21	Mask size 0 or 1 in LR			x	
22	Needle Cutter /Burner in Facility		x	x	x
23	Electric Sterilizer OR Boiler OR Autoclave Machine in Facility		x	x	x
24	Yellow color coded container in LR		x	x	x
25	Red color coded container in LR		x	x	x
26	White color coded container in LR		x	x	x
	Availability of at least one:	Supplies - Consumables			
27	Cap in LR		x	x	x
28	Apron in LR		x	x	x
29	Face Mask in LR		x	x	x
30	Chromic Catgut – No. 1 with round body needle in LR		x		
31	Gauze rolls (any size) in Facility		x	x	
32	Sanitary Pad (disposable) in Facility		x		
33	Intravenous Cannula 16G/18G/20G/22G/24G in Facility		x		
34	Foley's catheter (16) in Facility		x		
35	Mucus Sucker (Dee Lee's Type) in LR			x	
36	Cord clamp in LR			x	

·Continued

Sl. No.	Indicators	Domains	Service-specific readiness		
			Management of normal deliveries and emergency management of PPH	Newborn care (including management of asphyxia)	Infection prevention
	Availability of any stock-in quantity of:				
37	ANY uterotonic in the LR (oxytocin, misoprostol, methyldopa)	Supplies - Drugs	x		
38	Gel Lignocaine (2% or 5%), Injection Lignocaine/ Lidocaine (2% or 5% vial) in Facility		x		
39	Povidone Iodine (5% Betadine) Solution in Facility		x		x
40	Ringer Lactate (500 ml/ 1000 ml) in Facility		x		
41	20 IU Oxytocin in Facility**		x		
42	Injection Magnesium Sulphate (500 mg/ml ampoule) in Facility		x		
43	Availability of ANY hypertensive: Injection Labetalol (any strength), Capsule Nifedipine (5 mg) in Facility		x		
44	Availability of ANY Antibiotic in any strength: Capsule Amoxicillin, Injection Amoxicillin, Capsule Ampicillin, Injection Ampicillin, Injection Ceftriaxone, Inj. Amikacin, Injection Gentamycin in Facility		x	x	

Note: Positive Indicators were scored as 1 for 'yes' and 0 for 'no'; Negative Indicators were scored as 0 for 'yes' and 1 for 'no'

Legends: ANM: auxiliary nurse midwives; GNM: general nurse midwives; OBGYN: Obstetrician & Gynecologist; LR: Labor Room; PPH: postpartum hemorrhage

**Availability of at least 20 IU Oxytocin in the facility was separately awarded a score (in addition to "presence of any uterotonics") since this is the minimum loading dose required to start the treatment for PPH

2.2.2.3 Analysis of the facility readiness scores

Each assessed health facility received a facility readiness score for each of the CFAs, and the facilities could be matched based on their unique identifier (ID's) which were constant for a facility during any CFA. It was decided to consider the common facilities across CFA 2015, 2017 and 2019 to develop an understanding of the progress at 2-year intervals. A dataset of 524 ID-matched facilities was created, and the mean, median, minimum, and maximum facility readiness scores were compared separately for Level 2 and Level 3 facilities (summary changes) between the 3 CFAs. Hypothesis testing was conducted with paired t test for the mean change in scores, separately for each level, and separately for CFA 2017 vs. 2015 and CFA 2019 vs. 2017. A two-sided p-value <0.05 was considered to be significant. The degree of change (negative, no change or positive change) was also assessed for Level 2 and Level 3 facilities, separately for CFA 2017 vs. 2015 and CFA 2019 vs. 2017.

These 524 common facilities and their individual scores were next utilized to formulate the district-level readiness score – the score for each district representing the arithmetic mean of the facility readiness scores of all facilities (weighted equally) in that district. For example, if a district had 9 functional delivery points common across the 3 CFAs, the district-level readiness score was the arithmetic mean of the facility readiness scores of these 9 facilities, calculated separately for CFA 2015, 2017 and 2019. The mean district-level readiness score was calculated for the 3 CFAs, and the mean change in scores was compared separately for CFA 2017 vs. 2015 and CFA 2019 vs. 2017 using paired t test. A two-sided p-value <0.05 was considered to be significant. One-way analysis of variance (ANOVA) was conducted to test whether the mean facility readiness scores based on CFA 2015, 2017 and 2019 were significantly different from each other – separately for Level 2 and Level 3 facilities. Further, the trend in the facility readiness scores for each district over the 3 CFAs was anlayzed to identify those with a

continuously increasing score or otherwise. These trend categories were utilized to pictorially

depict the changes across the districts of Bihar using a heat map.

2.2.3 Ethical approval

The use of CFA data in this manuscript was determined as "not human subjects research" (under

45 CFR 46) by the Institutional Review Board at Columbia University, New York, USA

(Protocol #IRB-AAAT1461, decision dated June 20, 2020). The data generated through the

CFAs related to select facility-level characteristics like availability of human resources, physical

condition of the health facilities in terms of infrastructure, functionality of equipment and supply

of drugs and consumables. This data was retrospective, and also did not contain any individual-

level identifiers (non-human subject data).

2.3 Results

CFA 2017 involved assessing 476 Level 2 and 74 Level 3 delivery points (total 550 health

facilities), while 477 Level 2 and 75 Level 3 (total 552) delivery points were assessed during

CFA 2019. Over this period of time, one additional primary health center (Level 2 facility) was

functionalized in each of *Begusarai* and *East Champaran* districts, while one primary health

center in *Buxar* district became non-functional. The district hospital in Patna (Level 3 facility)

participated only during the 2019 CFA.

2.3.1 Comparative analysis of facility-level structural readiness: CFA 2017 vs. CFA 2019

Tables 2.1-2.9 demonstrates findings from the facility-level assessment of infrastructure, stock-

in status of essential supplies (equipment, drugs, consumables), human resources availability,

drug supply management, availability of ambulance services, laboratory service delivery, and

infection control and biomedical waste management practices. The detailed description of the findings in each of these distinct domains (like infrastructure, laboratory services etc.) has been provided in **Appendix B**, while a summary of the key findings is presented below.

2.3.1.1 Infrastructure

During both the 2017 and 2019 CFAs, at least 99% of Level 2 and Level 3 facilities provided 24x7 delivery services and had designated labor rooms, while at least 94% had designated maternity wards, drug-storage rooms, and laboratories. Among the Level 2 facilities, 97% had designated newborn care corners (NBCCs) during CFA 2019, and 82% of these were located inside labor rooms – an increase of about 6 percentage-points for both parameters. Among the Level 3 facilities, 97% had designated NBCCs and 88% of these were located inside labor rooms (minimal change from 2017 status). At both levels, notable improvements were observed in establishing handwashing stations (elbow taps with running water) in the labor rooms (67% at Level 2 (increased 15 percentage-points) and 85% at Level 3 (increased 29 percentage-points)) with simultaneous improvement in the availability of soap at these stations (increased 6 percentage-points at Level 2 and increased 21-points at Level 3). Despite an increase from 2017, only 22% of Level 2 and 13% of Level 3 facilities had an adequate number of labor tables as per RMNCH+A program specifications during CFA 2019, and only 72% of Level 2 (increased 41 percentage-points) and 80% of Level 3 (increased 66 percentage-points) facilities ensured proper spacing (at least 100 sq ft. area) between these tables.

During both assessments, about one-third of all facilities exhibited some signs of infrastructural damage (like water seepage) in their labor rooms, and there was lack of notable improvement in the physical condition of the maternity wards and laboratories. In contrast, improvements were noted in the condition of the drug-storage rooms – the proportion of such rooms having plastered brick walls increased 35 percentage-points among Level 2 facilities, and those having concrete roofs increased 88 percentage-points among Level 2 facilities, and increased 92 percentage-points among Level 3 facilities.

Table 2.1: Changes in the facility-level infrastructure, CFA 2017 vs. CFA 2019

	Level 2 health facilities					Level 3 health facilities				
	CFA 2017 (n=476)		CFA 2019 (n=477)		Change (% points)	CFA 2017 (n=74)		CFA 2019 (n=75)		Change (% points)
	n	%	n	%		n	%	n	%	
Labor room (LR)										
Facility provides 24X7 delivery services **(among all facilities)**	474	100%	474	99%	0%	74	100%	74	99%	-1%
Facility has a designated Labor room	**475**	100%	**476**	100%	0%	**74**	100%	**75**	100%	0%
Presence of toilet inside/within 1 meter of the LR	330	69%	358	75%	6%	51	69%	55	73%	4%
LRs have enough labor tables as specified in Maternal and Newborn Health toolkit	56	12%	103	22%	10%	5	7%	10	13%	7%
Sufficient LR area as per total available LR tables (100 sq ft. area required for each LR table)	149	31%	344	72%	41%	10	14%	60	80%	66%
Facility has Newborn Care Corner (NBCC, among all facilities)	434	91%	462	97%	6%	73	99%	73	97%	-1%
NBCC located inside labor room *(among those with NBCC)*	328	76%	381	82%	7%	65	89%	64	88%	-1%
All walls made of brick	472	99%	466	98%	-1%	74	100%	75	100%	0%
Brick walls with 6 ft. tiles (among facilities with brick walls)	72	15%	100	21%	6%	19	26%	28	37%	12%
Presence of cracks (at least 1 feet) on any wall	32	7%	54	11%	5%	3	4%	4	5%	1%
Signs of water seepage from any wall	185	39%	149	31%	-8%	27	36%	20	27%	-10%
Roof is made of concrete	464	98%	464	97%	0%	72	97%	72	96%	-1%
Sign of water seepage from the roof	152	32%	126	26%	-6%	17	23%	17	23%	0%
Sign of water seepage from wall and roof (both)	117	25%	97	20%	-4%	14	19%	13	17%	-2%
Floors with tiles or plastered	433	91%	442	93%	2%	67	91%	70	93%	3%
Can read a newspaper with available illumination	466	98%	465	98%	0%	73	99%	74	99%	0%
LR has back-up power supply (generator and/or invertor)	474	100%	475	100%	0%	74	100%	74	99%	-1%
Above, but no connection to radiant warmer	12	3%	23	5%	2%	0	0%	1	1%	1%
Above, but no connection to focus light	83	18%	109	23%	5%	8	11%	14	19%	8%

Continued

	Level 2 health facilities					Level 3 health facilities				
	CFA 2017 (n=476)		CFA 2019 (n=477)		Change (% points)	CFA 2017 (n=74)		CFA 2019 (n=75)		Change (% points)
	n	%	n	%		n	%	n	%	
Above, but no connection to oxygen concentrator	27	6%	37	8%	2%	4	5%	8	11%	5%
Above, but no connection to phototherapy	69	15%	122	26%	11%	11	15%	23	31%	16%
Above, but no connection to suction machine	59	12%	81	17%	5%	6	8%	11	15%	7%
Refrigerator available in LR	325	68%	324	68%	0%	55	74%	59	79%	4%
Presence of Elbow tap with running water in LR	245	52%	318	67%	15%	42	57%	64	85%	29%
Presence of normal tap with running water in LR	159	33%	102	21%	-12%	24	32%	6	8%	-24%
Soap available at handwashing station	415	87%	355	75%	-13%	62	84%	58	77%	-6%
Nothing available (soap or any spirit or sanitizers) at handwashing station	46	10%	87	18%	9%	8	11%	10	13%	3%
Elbow tap and soap (both available)	220	46%	247	52%	6%	35	47%	51	68%	21%
Maternity ward (MW) and associated Nursing Station										
Presence of designated maternity ward	**460**	97%	**448**	94%	-3%	**72**	97%	**74**	99%	1%
Facilities with 2 or more maternity wards (**among all facilities**)	149	31%	121	25%	-6%	54	73%	50	67%	-6%
Mean number of beds in maternity wards per facility	7.2		6.8			19.6		17.8		
Brick walls with 6 ft. tiles (at least 1 MW)	309	67%	249	56%	-12%	60	83%	55	74%	-9%
Presence of cracks (at least 1 feet) on any wall (in any MW)	33	7%	59	13%	6%	8	11%	13	18%	6%
Signs of water seepage from any wall (in any MW)	174	38%	99	22%	-16%	33	46%	24	32%	-13%
Sign of water seepage from the roof (any MW)	138	30%	112	25%	-5%	30	42%	24	32%	-9%
Floors with tiles or plastered (any MW)	356	77%	357	80%	2%	51	71%	58	78%	8%
MW has a toilet inside (any MW)	153	33%	153	34%	1%	20	28%	25	34%	6%
MW has a toilet facility just outside the ward (within 10 meters) (any MW)	210	46%	285	64%	18%	47	65%	60	81%	16%
MW has a toilet facility inside/just outside the wards (any MW)	338	73%	313	70%	-4%	61	85%	63	85%	0%

Continued

	Level 2 health facilities					Level 3 health facilities				
	CFA 2017 (n=476)		CFA 2019 (n=477)		Change (% points)	CFA 2017 (n=74)		CFA 2019 (n=75)		Change (% points)
	n	%	n	%		n	%	n	%	
MW has a power backup system (any MW)	456	99%	440	98%	-1%	72	100%	74	100%	0%
Can read a newspaper with available illumination (any MW)	450	98%	442	99%	1%	71	99%	74	100%	1%
Nursing station present (within or outside the MW)	413	90%	419	94%	4%	66	92%	67	91%	-1%
Handwashing station present inside the nursing station	180	39%	176	39%	0%	25	35%	25	34%	-1%
Dedicated toilet available inside the nursing station	146	32%	262	58%	27%	20	28%	44	59%	32%
Designated Kangaroo mother care corner/ area in the health facility **(among all facilities)**	no data		183	38%		no data		37	49%	
KMC corner/ area located within 10 meters from the Labor room (among all facilities)			154	32%				23	31%	
KMC corner/ area is a separate room or a demarcated space within a room with curtains (among all facilities)			122	26%				29	39%	
At least one bed available for mother to do feeding (among all facilities)			164	34%				32	43%	
Stool/Chair for the attendant (among all facilities)	53	11%	77	16%	5%	14	19%	15	20%	1%
Side screens (among all facilities)	171	36%	98	21%	-15%	16	22%	11	15%	-7%
IV Stands (among all facilities)	338	71%	329	69%	-2%	58	78%	59	79%	0%
Public display of communication material: (among all facilities)										
Danger signs for mother	207	43%	159	33%	-10%	39	53%	19	25%	-27%
Danger signs for new born	198	42%	136	29%	-13%	37	50%	18	24%	-26%
Breast feeding	311	65%	295	62%	-3%	55	74%	46	61%	-13%
Post-natal care	249	52%	196	41%	-11%	39	53%	23	31%	-22%
Kangaroo Mother Care	295	62%	267	56%	-6%	44	59%	40	53%	-6%
Family Planning Information	242	51%	235	49%	-2%	42	57%	35	47%	-10%

Continued

	Level 2 health facilities					Level 3 health facilities				
	CFA 2017 (n=476)		CFA 2019 (n=477)		Change (% points)	CFA 2017 (n=476)		CFA 2019 (n=477)		Change (% points)
	n	%	n	%		n	%	n	%	
Drug storage room										
Designated drug store	**469**	99%	**470**	99%	0%	72	97%	74	99%	1%
In any of the drug storage rooms:										
Brick walls plastered and/ or whitewashed	1	0.2%	163	35%	34%	3	4%	16	22%	17%
Cracks on any of the brick walls (1 ft or more long)	64	14%	119	25%	12%	10	14%	15	20%	6%
Signs of water seepage on any of the brick walls	193	41%	187	40%	-1%	31	43%	31	42%	-1%
Concrete roof in at least one room	4	0.9%	419	89%	88%	2	3%	70	95%	92%
Signs of water seepage from roof in at least one room	171	36%	174	37%	1%	29	40%	25	34%	-6%
At least one drug storage room has seepage in both wall & roof	143	30%	137	29%	-1%	23	32%	19	26%	-6%
Floor is cemented with tiles/ marble	0	0%	313	67%	67%	0	0%	48	65%	65%
Laboratory										
Facility has a designated Laboratory	**450**	95%	**457**	96%	1%	74	100%	74	99%	-1%
Lab provides 24*7 services	2	0.4%	5	1%	1%	5	7%	11	15%	8%
Elbow tap with running water	11	2%	14	3%	1%	7	9%	10	14%	4%
Normal tap with running water	306	68%	304	67%	-1%	56	76%	47	64%	-12%
Soap/ liquid soap available for hand washing	312	69%	290	63%	-6%	55	74%	47	64%	-11%
Alcohol-based solutions/ spirits available for hand washing	44	10%	43	9%	0%	12	16%	8	11%	-5%
Personal Protective Equipment (PPE) for lab technician: Masks	174	39%	194	42%	4%	33	45%	26	35%	-9%
PPE for lab technician: Aprons	138	31%	124	27%	-4%	29	39%	24	32%	-7%
PPE for lab technician: Gloves	323	72%	300	66%	-6%	53	72%	53	72%	0%
PPE for lab technician: Caps	27	6%	25	5%	-1%	6	8%	7	9%	1%
PPE for lab technician: Goggles	22	5%	27	6%	1%	6	8%	7	9%	1%
Laboratory has power back-up	417	93%	425	93%	0%	71	96%	66	89%	-7%

Note: All percentages are calculated based on the number of "designated" areas, unless mentioned otherwise

2.3.1.2 Essential supplies (equipment, drugs and consumables)

The supply chain system worked well to ensure that during CFA 2019, about 70% of facilities at either level had at least one functional fetal doppler (increased 5 percentage-points at Level 2), over 90% had digital or manual infant weighing machines, at least 84% had radiant warmers (increased at least 5 percentage-points at both levels), and over 80% had AMBU bags (artificial manual breathing units) with neonatal oxygen masks for resuscitation (increased 4 percentage-points at Level 3). However, the availability of a number of essential equipment like stethoscopes decreased by 11 percentage-points (from 72% in 2017), blood pressure machines decreased 16 percentage-points (from 76%), at least one of functional autoclave machine or electric sterilizer or boiler decreased 25 percentage-points (from 76%) and functional oxygen cylinders decreased 32 percentage-points (from 69%) deteriorated in the Level 2 facilities during CFA 2019. Level 3 facilities mirrored these changes.

The availability of different drugs in the labor rooms remained stable or improved between 2017 and 2019. Oxytocin was available in over 65% Level 2 or Level 3 facilities, Misoprostol in about 60% facilities (increased 13 percentage-points at Level 2 and decreased 9 percentage-points at Level 3), and magnesium sulphate in 67% of Level 2 (increased 7 percentage-points) and 77% of Level 3 (increased 6 percentage-points) facilities. Improvements were noted in the supply of vitamin K injections, antibiotics (Ampicillin and Gentamycin) and antihypertensives (Nifedipine tablets) by 7-32 percentage-points at both levels. Reproductive health supplies like condoms were available in 80% of Level 3 (increased 39 percentage-points) and 66% of Level 2 (decreased 4 percentage-points) facilities, intrauterine contraceptive devices (IUCD-375) were available in 57% Level 3 (increased 14 percentage-points) and 65% Level 2 (increased 30 percentage-points) facilities, sanitary napkins in 53% Level 3 (increased 15 percentage-points) and54% Level 2 (increased 21 percentage-points) facilities, iron and folic acid tablets were available in 41% of Level 2 (increased 11 percentage-points) and 47% of Level 3 (increased 5 percentage-points) facilities, and oral/ emergency contraceptives were available in 60% of Level 2 facilities and in at least 75% of Level 3 (increased about 40 percentage-points) facilities. In contrast, almost all facilities suffered from stock-out of Salbutamol, Labetalol, Methyldopa, normal saline and Ringer's lactate solutions. There was also deterioration in the supply of basic consumables like cotton and gauze rolls, intravenous cannulas and syringes, and urinary catheters and collection bags.

Table 2.2: Changes in the facility-level availability of at least one functional equipment on the day of visit, CFA 2017 vs. CFA 2019

	Level 2 health facilities					Level 3 health facilities				
	CFA 2017 (n=476)		CFA 2019 (n=4t66t77)		Change (% points)	CFA 2017 (n=74)		CFA 2019 (n=75)		Change (% points)
	n	%	n	%		n	%	n	%	
In the labor room										
Facilities with designated Labor rooms	475		476			74		75		
Stethoscope	342	72%	290	61%	-11%	58	78%	48	64%	-14%
BP apparatus (mercury)	246	52%	204	43%	-9%	44	59%	38	51%	-9%
BP apparatus (digital)	120	25%	98	21%	-5%	18	24%	15	20%	-4%
BP Apparatus (Mercury or Digital)	363	76%	287	60%	-16%	57	77%	47	63%	-14%
Fetal Doppler	310	65%	335	70%	5%	49	66%	51	68%	2%
Fetoscope	273	57%	249	52%	-5%	46	62%	30	40%	-22%
Mayo's trolley	238	50%	232	49%	-1%	41	55%	41	55%	-1%
Crash Cart	93	20%	137	29%	9%	22	30%	41	55%	25%
Autoclave Machine	302	64%	186	39%	-25%	43	58%	27	36%	-22%
Sterilization drum	400	84%	382	80%	-4%	66	89%	65	87%	-3%
Electric Sterilizer / Boiler	218	46%	122	26%	-20%	38	51%	15	20%	-31%
Digital Baby Weighing machine	381	80%	389	82%	2%	58	78%	65	87%	8%
Mechanical baby weighing machine	309	65%	218	46%	-19%	48	65%	33	44%	-21%
Digital or Manual baby weighing machine	465	98%	452	95%	-3%	69	93%	70	93%	0%
Ampoule cutter	49	10%	32	7%	-4%	10	14%	4	5%	-8%
Hub Cutter	238	50%	253	53%	3%	45	61%	46	61%	1%
Needle Cutter/Burner	116	24%	96	20%	-4%	24	32%	25	33%	1%
Pulse oximeter	85	18%	92	19%	1%	18	24%	24	32%	8%
Room Thermometer	147	31%	154	32%	1%	32	43%	37	49%	6%
Ambu bag (250 ml)	341	72%	364	76%	5%	48	65%	57	76%	11%
Ambu bag (500 ml)	259	55%	296	62%	8%	40	54%	49	65%	11%
Ambu bag 250/500 ml	448	94%	436	92%	-3%	69	93%	72	96%	3%

Continued

	Level 2 health facilities					Level 3 health facilities				
	CFA 2017 (n=476)		CFA 2019 (n=477)		Change (% points)	CFA 2017 (n=476)		CFA 2019 (n=477)		Change (% points)
	n	%	n	%		n	%	n	%	
Neonatal Mask - 0 size	317	67%	357	75%	8%	51	69%	61	81%	12%
Neonatal Mask - 1 size	298	63%	343	72%	9%	51	69%	54	72%	3%
Neonatal mask 0 OR 1 size	393	83%	402	84%	2%	62	84%	67	89%	6%
Neonatal mask 0 AND 1 size	222	47%	298	63%	16%	40	54%	48	64%	10%
AMBU Bag and Neonatal mask 0 OR 1 size	386	81%	391	82%	1%	61	82%	65	87%	4%
Clock	369	78%	372	78%	0%	64	86%	69	92%	6%
Haemoglobinometer	44	9%	69	14%	5%	9	12%	16	21%	9%
Foot operated suction machine	137	29%	122	26%	-3%	22	30%	22	29%	0%
Electric suction machine	no data		245	51%		no data		42	56%	
Stand Mobile Lamp/focus light	169	36%	178	37%	2%	31	42%	44	59%	17%
Emergency Light torch	55	12%	44	9%	-2%	9	12%	10	13%	1%
Foot steps	419	88%	443	93%	5%	73	99%	70	93%	-5%
Radiant Warmer	376	79%	399	84%	5%	64	86%	69	92%	6%
Phototherapy machine	no data		218	46%		no data		14	19%	
Oxygen Cylinder	329	69%	176	37%	-32%	55	74%	27	36%	-38%
Oxygen Cylinder with attached Flowmeter and humidifier	304	64%	283	59%	-5%	47	64%	44	59%	-5%
Oxygen concentrator	315	66%	300	63%	-3%	40	54%	46	61%	7%
Fetal Doppler/Fetoscope	384	81%	378	79%	-1%	59	80%	56	75%	-5%
Autoclave/ Electric Sterilizer /Boiler (at least one)	363	76%	243	51%	-25%	57	77%	34	45%	-32%

Continued

	Level 2 health facilities					Level 3 health facilities				
	CFA 2017 (n=476)		CFA 2019 (n=477)		Change (% points)	CFA 2017 (n=476)		CFA 2019 (n=477)		Change (% points)
	n	%	n	%		n	%	n	%	
In the maternity ward and associated nursing station										
Facilities with designated maternity wards	460		448			72		74		
BP apparatus (Mercury)	217	47%	215	48%	1%	33	46%	35	47%	1%
BP apparatus (Digital)	120	26%	131	29%	3%	12	17%	15	20%	4%
Stethoscopes	263	57%	269	60%	3%	40	56%	42	57%	1%
Fetoscope	97	21%	116	26%	5%	21	29%	21	28%	-1%
Fetal Doppler	121	26%	170	38%	12%	25	35%	26	35%	0%
Emergency Medicine Tray	51	11%	52	12%	1%	14	19%	11	15%	-5%
Sim's Speculum	160	35%	72	16%	-19%	25	35%	14	19%	-16%
Sponge holding forceps	172	37%	86	19%	-18%	26	36%	12	16%	-20%
Crash Cart	24	5%	19	4%	-1%	6	8%	7	9%	1%
Oxygen cylinder with all accessories (Flowmeter, Humidifier, Mask)	56	12%	48	11%	-1%	14	19%	9	12%	-7%
Oxygen cylinder (filled)	86	19%	59	13%	-6%	18	25%	10	14%	-11%
Wrench / Key	84	18%	59	13%	-5%	13	18%	11	15%	-3%
Anterior vaginal wall retractor	71	15%	27	6%	-9%	7	10%	4	5%	-4%
In the laboratory										
Facilities with designated Laboratories	450		457			74		74		
Semi-Auto analyzer	358	80%	318	70%	-10%	70	95%	57	77%	-18%
Auto-Analyzer	20	4%	46	10%	6%	11	15%	11	15%	0%
Hemoglobin meter	382	85%	379	83%	-2%	67	91%	62	84%	-7%
Centrifuge	294	65%	312	68%	3%	63	85%	59	80%	-5%
Refrigerator	241	54%	265	58%	4%	63	85%	63	85%	0%
Incubator	182	40%	194	42%	2%	44	59%	42	57%	-3%

Continued

	Level 2 health facilities					Level 3 health facilities				
	CFA 2017 (n=476)		CFA 2019 (n=477)		Change (% points)	CFA 2017 (n=476)		CFA 2019 (n=477)		Change (% points)
	n	%	n	%		n	%	n	%	
Elisa Reader	9	2%	6	1%	-1%	3	4%	4	5%	1%
ESR stand	167	37%	172	38%	1%	55	74%	54	73%	-1%
Binocular Microscope	348	77%	311	68%	-9%	54	73%	49	66%	-7%
Monocular Microscope	39	9%	47	10%	2%	22	30%	19	26%	-4%
Hub Cutter	76	17%	110	24%	7%	35	47%	39	53%	5%
Syringe and Needle Destroyer/terminator	32	7%	54	12%	5%	18	24%	18	24%	0%

Note: All percentages are calculated based on the number of "designated" areas, unless mentioned otherwise

Table 2.3: Changes in the facility-level availability of any stock-in quantity of a consumable on the day of visit, CFA 2017 vs. CFA 2019

	Level 2 health facilities					Level 3 health facilities				
	CFA 2017 (n=476)		CFA 2019 (n=477)		Change (% points)	CFA 2017 (n=74)		CFA 2019 (n=75)		Change (% points)
	n	%	n	%		n	%	n	%	
In the labor room										
Facilities with designated Labor rooms	475		476			74		75		
Absorbent Gauze	352	74%	325	68%	-6%	59	80%	51	68%	-12%
Cap	245	52%	259	54%	3%	40	54%	45	60%	6%
Apron	410	86%	410	86%	0%	62	84%	63	84%	0%
Face Mask	346	73%	340	71%	-1%	56	76%	59	79%	3%
cap, mask, apron (all)	213	45%	222	47%	2%	37	50%	37	49%	-1%
Chromic Catgut	290	61%	275	58%	-3%	38	51%	46	61%	10%
Cord Clamp	346	73%	407	86%	13%	49	66%	64	85%	19%
Cotton	441	93%	360	76%	-17%	68	92%	55	73%	-19%
Foley's Catheter	309	65%	270	57%	-8%	57	77%	40	53%	-24%
Uro bag	185	39%	219	46%	7%	41	55%	47	63%	7%
Foley's catheter and uro bag (both)	163	34%	39	8%	-26%	39	53%	7	9%	-43%
HIV Testing Kit	169	36%	144	30%	-5%	32	43%	36	48%	5%
Bleaching powder	416	88%	362	76%	-12%	64	86%	59	79%	-8%
Condom	333	70%	316	66%	-4%	30	41%	60	80%	39%
IUCD 375	167	35%	309	65%	30%	32	43%	43	57%	14%
IUCD 380A	352	74%	237	50%	-24%	53	72%	44	59%	-13%
IUCD (380A or 375)	417	88%	393	83%	-5%	65	88%	67	89%	1%
IV Cannula 18G	137	29%	153	32%	3%	30	41%	25	33%	-7%
IV Cannula 20G	182	38%	154	32%	-6%	35	47%	33	44%	-3%
IV Cannula 22G	158	33%	137	29%	-4%	36	49%	25	33%	-15%

Continued

	Level 2 health facilities					Level 3 health facilities				
	CFA 2017 (n=476)		CFA 2019 (n=477)		Change (% points)	CFA 2017 (n=74)		CFA 2019 (n=75)		Change (% points)
	n	%	n	%		n	%	n	%	
IV Cannula 24G	95	20%	99	21%	1%	14	19%	18	24%	5%
any cannula	335	71%	312	66%	-5%	64	86%	56	75%	-12%
Mucus Sucker (Dee Lee's Type)	342	72%	340	71%	-1%	56	76%	54	72%	-4%
Povidone Iodine Solution	397	84%	360	76%	-8%	64	86%	60	80%	-6%
Pregnancy Test Kits (Nischay Kit)	131	28%	116	24%	-3%	7	9%	8	11%	1%
Sanitary Napkin (Pad)	155	33%	255	54%	21%	28	38%	40	53%	15%
Suction Tube	271	57%	275	58%	1%	39	53%	41	55%	2%
Surgical Spirit	272	57%	232	49%	-9%	54	73%	46	61%	-12%
Syringe 1 ml	66	14%	103	22%	8%	19	26%	13	17%	-8%
Syringe 2 ml	245	52%	248	52%	1%	39	53%	35	47%	-6%
Syringe 5 ml	366	77%	361	76%	-1%	60	81%	62	83%	2%
Syringe 10ml	241	51%	274	58%	7%	44	59%	48	64%	5%
Syringe 20 ml	39	8%	95	20%	12%	6	8%	22	29%	21%
0.1ml AD syringe with needle	204	43%	137	29%	-14%	22	30%	17	23%	-7%
0.5ml AD syringe with needle	225	47%	154	32%	-15%	26	35%	20	27%	-8%
any syringe	429	90%	426	89%	-1%	65	88%	69	92%	4%
Cotton Thread	310	65%	247	52%	-13%	36	49%	28	37%	-11%
Towel for New born Baby	231	49%	229	48%	-1%	41	55%	31	41%	-14%
Gown for patient in labor	78	16%	85	18%	1%	16	22%	19	25%	4%
Macintosh Sheet on all Labor table	306	64%	357	75%	11%	50	68%	53	71%	3%
In the maternity ward and associated Nursing Station										
Facilities with designated Maternity wards	460		448			72		74		
Cotton rolls (Any Size)	298	65%	138	31%	-34%	46	64%	23	31%	-33%
Gauze rolls (Any Size)	264	57%	124	28%	-30%	42	58%	13	18%	-41%

Continued

	Level 2 health facilities					Level 3 health facilities				
	CFA 2017 (n=476)		CFA 2019 (n=477)		Change (% points)	CFA 2017 (n=74)		CFA 2019 (n=75)		Change (% points)
	n	%	n	%		n	%	n	%	
Gloves	258	56%	177	40%	-17%	44	61%	24	32%	-29%
Foley's catheter (16)	113	25%	68	15%	-9%	26	36%	16	22%	-14%
Nasogastric (Ryle's) tube	32	7%	21	5%	-2%	7	10%	4	5%	-4%
Intravenous Cannula (16)	13	3%	25	6%	3%	1	1%	1	1%	0%
Intravenous Cannula (18)	79	17%	45	10%	-7%	13	18%	6	8%	-10%
Intravenous Cannula (20)	112	24%	58	13%	-11%	24	33%	12	16%	-17%
Intravenous Cannula (22)	102	22%	42	9%	-13%	29	40%	10	14%	-27%
Intravenous Cannula (24)	64	14%	42	9%	-5%	10	14%	7	9%	-4%
Sanitary Pad (Disposable)	84	18%	63	14%	-4%	17	24%	15	20%	-3%
Syringe (10ml)	143	31%	96	21%	-10%	28	39%	14	19%	-20%
Syringe (2ml)	142	31%	103	23%	-8%	13	18%	13	18%	0%
Syringe (5ml)	220	48%	162	36%	-12%	39	54%	25	34%	-20%
Uro bag	86	19%	75	17%	-2%	21	29%	14	19%	-10%
In the laboratory										
Facilities with designated Laboratories	450		457			74		74		
Pregnancy Testing Kit (Nischay Kit)	297	66%	337	74%	8%	48	65%	62	84%	19%
Anti A serum	162	36%	183	40%	4%	41	55%	46	62%	7%
Anti B serum	160	36%	183	40%	4%	41	55%	46	62%	7%
Anti RH serum	162	36%	181	40%	4%	42	57%	46	62%	5%
Copper Sulphate Solution (Hb %)	150	33%	298	65%	32%	27	36%	51	69%	32%
Anti-coagulants	154	34%	241	53%	19%	50	68%	46	62%	-5%
Glucose powder	138	31%	131	29%	-2%	38	51%	26	35%	-16%
Reagents for GTT (used in Semi-Auto analyzer)	169	38%	164	36%	-2%	46	62%	30	41%	-22%
Urine Dipstick	279	62%	316	69%	7%	56	76%	57	77%	1%
VDRL Kit	229	51%	202	44%	-7%	37	50%	33	45%	-5%

Continued

	Level 2 health facilities					Level 3 health facilities				
	CFA 2017 (n=476)		CFA 2019 (n=477)		Change (% points)		CFA 2017 (n=74)		CFA 2019 (n=75)		Change (% points)
	n	%	n	%		n	%	n	%	
Reagents for Serum Urea and Creatinine	122	27%	162	35%	8%	42	57%	51	69%	12%
Rapid Testing Kit for Malaria	294	65%	387	85%	19%	44	59%	66	89%	30%
Rapid Kit 39 (RK-39) for Kala-Azar	318	71%	302	66%	-5%	53	72%	51	69%	-3%
HIV testing Kit	424	94%	435	95%	1%	60	81%	65	88%	7%
HBV testing Kit	146	32%	173	38%	5%	35	47%	46	62%	15%
Personal Protective Equipment (PPE) for lab technician: Masks	174	39%	194	42%	4%	33	45%	26	35%	-9%
PPE for lab technician: Aprons	138	31%	124	27%	-4%	29	39%	24	32%	-7%
PPE for lab technician: Gloves	323	72%	300	66%	-6%	53	72%	53	72%	0%
PPE for lab technician: Caps	27	6%	25	5%	-1%	6	8%	7	9%	1%
PPE for lab technician: Goggles	22	5%	27	6%	1%	6	8%	7	9%	1%

Note: All percentages are calculated based on the number of "designated" areas, unless mentioned otherwise

Table 2.4: Changes in the facility-level availability of any stock-in quantity of a drug on the day of visit, CFA 2017 vs. CFA 2019

	Level 2 health facilities					Level 3 health facilities				
	CFA 2017 (n=476)		CFA 2019 (n=477)		Change (% points)	CFA 2017 (n=74)		CFA 2019 (n=75)		Change (% points)
	n	%	n	%		n	%	n	%	
In the labor room										
Facilities with designated Labor rooms	475		476			74		75		
Injection Oxytocin (any strength)	329	69%	324	68%	-1%	51	69%	50	67%	-2%
Injection Magnesium Sulphate (any strength)	282	59%	318	67%	7%	53	72%	58	77%	6%
Injection Vitamin K 1 (Phytonadione)	186	39%	252	53%	14%	36	49%	42	56%	7%
Injection Gentamycin (any strength)	254	53%	221	46%	-7%	30	41%	43	57%	17%
Salbutamol nebulizing solution Bottle	3	0.6%	2	0%	0%	0	0%	0	0%	0%
Syrup Salbutamol (2mg/5ml) bottle	2	0.4%	0	0%	0%	0	0%	0	0%	0%
Tablet Misoprostol (200 mcg)	232	49%	293	62%	13%	49	66%	43	57%	-9%
Tab. Methyl Dopa 250 mg	4	0.8%	2	0%	0%	0	0%	0	0%	0%
Tab Labetalol 100mg	1	0.2%	4	1%	1%	0	0%	1	1%	1%
Inj Labetalol	0	0%	1	0%	0%	1	1%	2	3%	1%
Tablet Zinc Sulphate dispersible	16	3%	25	5%	2%	2	3%	1	1%	-1%
Cap Nifedipine (5 mg)	76	16%	126	26%	10%	15	20%	21	28%	8%
Tab Iron folic acid (large or small)	143	30%	194	41%	11%	31	42%	35	47%	5%
Tablet folic acid 400 mcg	4	0.8%	2	0%	0%	1	1%	0	0%	-1%
Inj. Ampicillin (500 mg) vial	81	17%	158	33%	16%	7	9%	31	41%	32%
Capsule Ampicillin (any strength)	40	8%	51	11%	2%	5	7%	4	5%	-1%
Tab Metronidazole 400mg	245	52%	234	49%	-2%	28	38%	27	36%	-2%
Inj. Amoxicillin (any strength)	17	4%	26	5%	2%	3	4%	4	5%	1%
Cap. Amoxicillin (any strength)	130	27%	68	14%	-13%	19	26%	11	15%	-11%

Continued

	Level 2 health facilities					Level 3 health facilities				
	CFA 2017 (n=476)		CFA 2019 (n=477)		Change (% points)	CFA 2017 (n=74)		CFA 2019 (n=75)		Change (% points)
	n	%	n	%		n	%	n	%	
Inj. Ceftriaxone (any strength)	104	22%	81	17%	-5%	24	32%	22	29%	-3%
Tablet Paracetamol 500mg	275	58%	258	54%	-4%	32	43%	28	37%	-6%
Oral contraceptive pills (MALA-N)	281	59%	285	60%	1%	26	35%	60	80%	45%
Emergency contraceptive pills (I-pill)	252	53%	278	58%	5%	28	38%	57	76%	38%
Inj. Calcium Gluconate (10 mg/ml)	77	16%	139	29%	13%	16	22%	28	37%	16%
Injection Lignocaine/ Lidocaine (2% vials)	no data		250	53%		no data		38	51%	
Injection Lignocaine/lidocaine (5% vials)			5	1%				1	1%	
Gel Lignocaine (2% or 5%)			61	13%				7	9%	
In the maternity ward and associated Nursing Station										
Facilities with designated Maternity wards	460		448			72		74		
Betadine (Povidone Iodine)	206	45%	103	23%	-22%	35	49%	18	24%	-24%
Chlorhexidine Gluconate + Cetrimide (Savlon) in liters	128	28%	37	8%	-20%	21	29%	9	12%	-17%
Dextrose 5% (any)	182	40%	93	21%	-19%	36	50%	17	23%	-27%
Normal Saline 100 ml bottle 0.9%	214	47%	8	2%	-45%	37	51%	0	0%	-51%
Ringer Lactate (500 or 1000 ml)_Any	234	51%	107	24%	-27%	41	57%	21	28%	-29%
Tablet Diclofenac	97	21%	32	7%	-14%	17	24%	4	5%	-18%
Tablet Paracetamol (500 mg)	206	45%	116	26%	-19%	30	42%	12	16%	-25%
Injection Gentamycin (80 mg/2ml or 40 mg/ml) (Vial/Ampoule)	150	33%	65	15%	-18%	27	38%	12	16%	-21%
Injection Ampicillin (500mg) (Vial)	42	9%	68	15%	6%	8	11%	10	14%	2%
Infusion Metronidazole (500mg/100ml) (Bottle)	101	22%	53	12%	-10%	18	25%	13	18%	-7%
Syrup Metronidazole (Bottle) (200mg/100ml)	5	1%	2	0.4%	-1%	0	0%	0	0%	0%
Tablet Metronidazole (400 mg)	170	37%	74	17%	-20%	23	32%	13	18%	-14%

Continued

	Level 2 health facilities					Level 3 health facilities				
	CFA 2017 (n=476)		CFA 2019 (n=477)		Change (% points)	CFA 2017 (n=74)		CFA 2019 (n=75)		Change (% points)
	n	%	n	%		n	%	n	%	
Tablet Misoprostol (200 mcg)	121	26%	93	21%	-6%	24	33%	16	22%	-12%
Inj. Adrenaline	60	13%	95	21%	8%	16	22%	18	24%	2%
Inj. Hydrocortisone Succinate	71	15%	67	15%	0%	21	29%	24	32%	3%
Inj. Dexamethasone	231	50%	168	38%	-13%	40	56%	36	49%	-7%
Inj. Aminophylline	51	11%	44	10%	-1%	9	13%	9	12%	0%

Note: All percentages are calculated based on the number of "designated" areas, unless mentioned otherwise

2.3.1.3 Human resources

Among all categories of health care providers, the availability of ANM nurses during both CFAs remained comparatively better – they were present at 57% of their sanctioned strength in Level 2 facilities during CFA 2019 (decreased 1 percentage-point from CFA 2017), and at 67% of their sanctioned strength in Level 3 facilities (increased 4 percentage-points from CFA 2017). However, a large number of contractually-hired ANMs were present at both levels during either CFAs. At Level 2 health facilities, 1416 such ANMs were available for service during CFA 2017 (thereby increasing the total number available for service to 3429 vs. sanctioned strength of 3479), while 2723 contractual ANMs were present during CFA 2019 (total number = 4606 vs. sanctioned strength of 3288). At Level 3 facilities, 122 contractual ANMs were present during CFA 2017 (total number = 290 vs. sanctioned strength of 270), and 191 were present during CFA 2019 (total number = 396 vs. sanctioned strength of 308).

In contrast, there were challenges in recruiting and/or retaining the GNM and physician cadres. During CFA 2019, the proportion of GNM nurses available for service decreased 29 percentage-points at Level 2 facilities (from 50% availability during CFA 2017), and decreased 2 percentage-points at Level 3 facilities (from 37% availability during CFA 2017). However, the number of contractually hired GNMs who were additionally available for service improved at both levels during CFA 2019 in comparison to CFA 2017 (Level 2: 144 vs. 61, Level 3: 33 vs. 0).

The availability of general-duty medical officers (primary care physicians) was 47% at Level 2 and 46% at Level 3 facilities during CFA 2019 – a deterioration by at least 8 percentage-points from CFA 2017. The number of contractually hired medical officers also decreased from 396 (CFA 2017) to 276 (CFA 2019) in Level 2 facilities, but remained constant at 44 in Level 3 facilities. This was somewhat counterbalanced by increased availability of internal medicine specialists at both levels – the numbers available increased more than 9 times at Level 2 and more than doubled at Level 3. The number of contractually hired internal medicine specialists also increased from 10 to 76 at Level 2 facilities, and from 16 to 36 at Level 3 facilities, over these 2 years.

During CFA 2019, the availability of general surgeons, OBGYNs, anesthesiologists and pediatricians deteriorated at Level 2 facilities (none were present in more than 20% of their sanctioned strength), but mostly improved across Level 3 facilities (available at around 40% of sanctioned strength, except for anesthesiologists at 28%). The numbers of contractually hired specialist physicians were insufficient to make any notable impact on the percentage available for service.

The additional data collected during 2019 showed ongoing efforts to recruit technicians, pharmacists, counsellors, data entry operators and clerical staff at both Level 2 and Level 3 facilities. However, a large number of such staff were recruited on a contractual basis – for example, 775 contractual data entry operators at Level 2 (vs. 62 regular recruitments) and 190 at Level 3 (vs. 17 regular recruitments) were additionally available for service. Similarly, a large number of contractually hired laboratory technicians (368 at Level 2 and 91 at Level 3) and counsellors (65 at Level 2 and 56 at Level 3) were also available during CFA 2019. Further, 270 (49%) out of 553 sanctioned positions for managerial staff – including block-level health managers, community mobilizers, monitoring and evaluation officers, account managers, and district health manager positions had been filled during CFA 2019. Additionally, 1505 such staff members had been contractually hired to support the implementation of the BTSP.

Table 2.5: Changes in the availability of human resources, CFA 2017 vs. CFA 2019

	Level 2 health facilities						Level 3 health facilities						
	CFA 2017 (n=476 facilities)			CFA 2019 (n=477 facilities)			Change (%points)	CFA 2017 (n=74 facilities)			CFA 2019 (n=75 facilities)			Change (% points)
	positions sanctioned	positions filled	%Available for service	positions sanctioned	positions filled	%Available for service		positions sanctioned	positions filled	%Available for service	positions sanctioned	positions filled	%Available for service	
General Duty Medical Officers	1967	1158	59%	1537	725	47%	-12%	694	378	54%	859	396	46%	-8%
Staff Nurse (GNM)	376	189	50%	831	174	21%	-29%	4575	1680	37%	4862	1675	34%	-2%
ANM nurses	3479	2013	58%	3288	1883	57%	-1%	270	168	62%	308	205	67%	4%
Specialist: Physician (Internal Medicine)	125	37	30%	812	356	44%	14%	161	61	38%	280	143	51%	13%
Specialist: General Surgeon	92	33	36%	120	22	18%	-18%	148	67	45%	158	74	47%	2%
Specialist: OBGYN	110	24	22%	118	23	19%	-2%	192	68	35%	209	81	39%	3%
Specialist: Anesthesiologist	71	7	10%	111	4	4%	-6%	153	45	29%	174	48	28%	-2%
Specialist: Pediatrician	86	17	20%	100	16	16%	-4%	149	58	39%	144	59	41%	2%
Laboratory Technicians	no data			586	90	15%		no data			362	72	20%	
Radiography Technicians				192	52	27%					236	98	42%	
Pharmacists				649	306	47%					356	169	47%	
Counsellors (RMNCH+A or Family Planning)				134	28	21%					37	9	24%	

Continued

	Level 2 health facilities							Level 3 health facilities						
	CFA 2017 (n=476 facilities)			CFA 2019 (n=477 facilities)			Change (% points)	CFA 2017 (n=74 facilities)			CFA 2019 (n=75 facilities)			Change (% points)
	positions sanctioned	positions filled	%Available for service	positions sanctioned	positions filled	%Available for service		positions sanctioned	positions filled	%Available for service	positions sanctioned	positions filled	%Available for service	
Data Entry Operators				173	62	36%					48	17	35%	
Clerical staff				965	735	76%					234	167	71%	
Block Health Manager				126	63	50%					12	5	42%	
Block Community Mobilizer	no data			125	62	50%		no data			2	1	50%	
Block Monitoring and Evaluation Officer				124	59	48%					2	0	0%	
Block Accounts Manager				134	74	55%					8	3	38%	
District Health Manager			not applicable								20	3	15%	

Note: Positions sanctioned: Total of positions that were sanctioned by Govt. of Bihar for each facility

Positions filled: Total of positions filled against the sanctioned positions

Available for service = # (filled through regular recruitment + deputation-in) - # (deputation-out + absent for 3 months), EXCLUDES all contractual employees

2.3.1.4 Other domains

The availability of functional ambulances as well as the referral transport service provision improved across both Level 2 and Level 3 facilities between CFA 2017 and 2019. 94% Level 2 (increased 15 percentage-points) and 99% Level 3 (increased 9 percentage-points) facilities had at least one functional ambulance during CFA 2019. In the 30 days prior to CFA 2019, the average number of pickups (from home to health facility) and drop-offs (for discharged mothers with newborn, from facility to home) per ambulance increased, compared to 2017. During this time period, the ambulances at Level 2 facilities traveled less distance (on average, CFA 2019 vs. 2017), likely indicating that referrals to a higher level facility occurred more frequently within the district. On the other hand, the average distance traveled by each ambulance increased at Level 3 facilities, as the journey likely involved transferring patients to another district hospital or to a medical college.

The laboratories across both levels of facilities benefitted from improved supply of reagents and chemicals, and could provide higher volume of services during CFA 2019 compared to CFA 2017. 74% Level 2 facilities (increased 8 percentage-points) and 84% Level 3 facilities (increased 19 percentage-points) with a designated laboratory had availability of pregnancy testing kits, while at least 85% facilities at either level had HIV and Malaria testing kits (increased at least 20 percentage-points), and 65% had reagents for hemoglobin estimation (increased 32 percentage-points at both levels). In the 30 days prior to CFA 2019, more than 90% of facilities with designated laboratories (at either level) conducted hemoglobin assessments and testing for malaria and HIV, 80% conducted urine pregnancy tests, and over 70% performed urinary glucose and albumin tests – representing an improvement by 10-60 percentage-points from CFA 2017.

Remarkable improvements were also noted in the use of web-based software (*e-Aushadhi*) to manage the facility-level drug-store inventories. During CFA 2019, the software was being used at 193 (41%) Level 2 (increased 40 percentage-points from CFA 2017) and 38 (51%) Level 3 (increased 46 percentage-points) facilities with designated drug storage rooms. Among the facilities where *e-Aushadhi* was being used, 80% (at either level) utilized this software for online indenting (i.e. placing request for supplies) to the district drug warehouse, but not so much for distribution of drugs to the different departments within the facility.

With regards to biomedical waste management, 91% of Level 2 (increased 7 percentage-points from CFA 2017) and 99% of Level 3 (increased 4 percentage-points) facilities were serviced by a professional agency during CFA 2019, though regular collection was documented in 60% Level 2 and 80% Level 3 facilities (both increased about 15 percentage-points). A total of 85% of facilities (at both levels) were reported to be preparing fresh 0.5 % hypochlorite solution every 24 hours – though only 60% facilities used this solution to clean the labor room floors and tables. Among the different colored containers for biomedical waste disposal, red (*for recyclable solid contaminated waste*) and yellow (*for anatomical waste, soiled waste, discarded medicines, laboratory waste, discarded contaminated linen & beddings etc.*) containers were present in at least 90%facilities at either level during CFA 2019. However, the white containers (*for waste sharps & metals*) were present in only 25% of Level 2 (increased 12 percentage-points) and 37% of Level 3 (increased 20 percentage-points) facilities, resulting in incorrect syringe disposal practices at most facilities. The disposal of gloves, dressing material, placenta, intravenous bottles and tubing were correctly done at over 80% of Level 2 and Level 3 facilities during both CFAs.

Table 2.6: Changes in the facility-level ambulance availability and service delivery, CFA 2017 vs. CFA 2019

	Level 2 health facilities					Level 3 health facilities				
	CFA 2017 (n=476)		CFA 2019 (n=477)		Change (% points)	CFA 2017 (n=74)		CFA 2019 (n=75)		Change (% points)
	n	%	n	%		n	%	n	%	
Total number of ambulances	633		687		54	222		242		20
Average number of ambulances per facility (mean)	1.3		1.4		0.1	2.9		3.2		0.3
Facility has an ambulance	459	96%	467	98%	1%	73	99%	75	100%	1%
At least one ambulance of the facility is functional (on road)	372	78%	446	94%	15%	66	89%	74	99%	9%
At least one ambulance of the facility is not functional (off road)	181	38%	112	23%	-15%	37	50%	30	40%	-10%
All ambulances of the facility are functional (on road)	278	58%	355	74%	16%	36	49%	45	60%	11%
A local contact number publicly available (for at least 1 ambulance)	271	57%	412	86%	29%	42	57%	67	89%	33%
All ambulances have registers	296	62%	374	78%	16%	43	58%	37	49%	-9%
For the last 30 days before CFA										
Average number of pick-ups per ambulance	51.9		57.5		5.6	19.9		30.2		10.3
Average number of drop-offs per ambulance	61.6		80.9		19.3	25.8		59.6		33.8
Average number of referrals to higher level facilities, per ambulance	11.1		18.9		7.8	12.1		15.4		3.3
Average distance travelled (km.), per ambulance	3790.1		2617.7		-1172.4	2232.5		3203.5		971.0

Table 2.7a: Changes in infection control, biomedical waste (BMW) management and management of condemned articles, CFA 2017 vs. CFA 2019

	Level 2 health facilities					Level 3 health facilities				
	CFA 2017 (n=476)		CFA 2019 (n=477)		Change (% points)	CFA 2017 (n=74)		CFA 2019 (n=75)		Change (% points)
	n	%	n	%		n	%	n	%	
Infection Control Practices in the labor room										
Facilities with designated Labor rooms	475		476			74		75		
Fresh 0.5 % hypochlorite solution made every 24 hours	403	85%	404	85%	0%	68	92%	64	85%	-7%
Labor room floor cleaned after each delivery	246	52%	294	62%	10%	31	42%	33	44%	2%
LR floor cleaned with hypochlorite solution	288	61%	252	53%	-8%	41	55%	44	59%	3%
LR floor cleaned with detergent/phenyl	236	50%	207	43%	-6%	47	64%	28	37%	-26%
Labor table cleaned after each delivery	448	94%	449	94%	0%	64	86%	69	92%	6%
Labor table cleaned with hypochlorite solution	303	64%	283	59%	-4%	46	62%	49	65%	3%
Labor table cleaned with detergent/phenyl	186	39%	137	29%	-10%	32	43%	13	17%	-26%
Cidex solution is available	174	37%	160	34%	-3%	29	39%	34	45%	6%
Needles recapped after use	237	50%	211	44%	-6%	33	45%	36	48%	3%
Needles burnt/cut in hub cutter before disposal	316	67%	351	74%	7%	51	69%	50	67%	-2%
BMW Management in the FACILITY (overall)										
Central collection point for BMW available	170	36%	178	37%	2%	38	51%	40	53%	2%
Any agency providing BMW management services to facility	398	84%	432	91%	7%	70	95%	74	99%	4%
Facility has register/card for recording/ monitoring BMW management services	189	40%	104	22%	-18%	42	57%	23	31%	-26%
Register with date and weight column available and completely filled	103	22%	52	11%	-11%	19	26%	11	15%	-11%
BMW collection is regular (once/day or alternate days)	210	44%	286	60%	16%	48	65%	60	80%	15%
Different colored liners sealed before dumping to central point or loading in truck and kept separately	233	49%	158	33%	-16%	40	54%	32	43%	-11%
Deep burial pits available in the facility campus	116	24%	153	32%	8%	17	23%	25	33%	10%

Continued

	Level 2 health facilities					Level 3 health facilities				
	CFA 2017 (n=476)		CFA 2019 (n=477)		Change (% points)	CFA 2017 (n=74)		CFA 2019 (n=75)		Change (% points)
	n	%	n	%		n	%	n	%	
Sharp pits available in the facility campus	123	26%	134	28%	2%	14	19%	23	31%	12%
No pits available in the facility campus	265	56%	226	47%	-8%	50	68%	40	53%	-14%
Facility has necessary permission from District Pollution Control Department for pits	111	23%	163	34%	11%	17	23%	22	29%	6%
Either BMW agency or BMW pits available with facility	425	89%	464	97%	8%	73	99%	74	99%	0%
Both BMW agency and any of BMW pits available with facility	184	39%	219	46%	7%	21	28%	35	47%	18%
No BMW agency or any pit available with facility	51	11%	13	3%	-8%	1	1%	1	1%	0%
Managing condemned articles in the facility (overall)										
Demarcated space for keeping condemned (junk) material	228	48%	311	65%	17%	47	64%	61	81%	18%
Where is the demarcated space?										
a) inside the building	113	24%	169	35%	12%	31	42%	45	60%	18%
b) outside the building	115	24%	192	40%	16%	16	22%	25	33%	12%
Is any condemned article present in the room										
a) Labor Room	24	5%	24	5%	0%	8	11%	8	11%	0%
b) OT	18	4%	36	8%	4%	13	18%	9	12%	-6%
c) Drug Store	77	16%	61	13%	-3%	15	20%	18	24%	4%
d) Maternity Ward	32	7%	17	4%	-3%	5	7%	6	8%	1%
e) Nursing Station	25	5%	25	5%	0%	2	3%	4	5%	3%
f) Pharmacy	31	7%	11	2%	-4%	6	8%	4	5%	-3%
g) Lab	43	9%	21	4%	-5%	5	7%	9	12%	5%
h) OPD	12	3%	11	2%	0%	3	4%	4	5%	1%
i) Corridor	136	29%	135	28%	0%	25	34%	33	44%	10%

Table 2.7b: Changes in biomedical waste (BMW) management practices in the labor room, CFA 2017 vs. CFA 2019

		Level 2 health facilities with designated LABOR ROOMS					Level 3 health facilities with designated LABOR ROOMS				
		CFA 2017 (n=475)		CFA 2019 (n=476)		Change (% points)	CFA 2017 (n=74)		CFA 2019 (n=75)		Change (% points)
		n	%	n	%		n	%	n	%	
Presence of color coded containers	Red containers present (recyclable solid contaminated waste)	427	90%	430	90%	0%	65	88%	72	96%	8%
	Red containers have same colored plastic bags	169	36%	166	35%	-1%	24	32%	30	40%	8%
	Red containers have 1% hypochlorite solution	168	35%	98	21%	-15%	24	32%	12	16%	-16%
	Yellow containers present (anatomical waste, soiled waste, discarded medicines, laboratory waste, discarded contaminated linen & beddings etc.)	438	92%	440	92%	0%	69	93%	74	99%	5%
	Yellow containers have same colored plastic bags	171	36%	176	37%	1%	38	51%	30	40%	-11%
	Yellow containers have 1% hypochlorite solution	157	33%	95	20%	-13%	24	32%	11	15%	-18%
	White containers present (waste sharps & metals)	62	13%	117	25%	12%	13	18%	28	37%	20%

Continued

		Level 2 health facilities with designated LABOR ROOMS					Level 3 health facilities with designated LABOR ROOMS				
		CFA 2017 (n=475)		CFA 2019 (n=476)		Change (% points)	CFA 2017 (n=74)		CFA 2019 (n=75)		Change (% points)
		n	%	n	%		n	%	n	%	
	White containers have same colored plastic bags	7	1%	0	0%	-1%	3	4%	0	0%	-4%
	White containers have 1% hypochlorite solution	29	6%	26	5%	-1%	4	5%	5	7%	1%
	Blue containers present (glassware)	67	14%	189	40%	26%	19	26%	43	57%	32%
	Blue containers have same colored plastic bags	8	2%	22	5%	3%	3	4%	2	3%	-1%
	Blue containers have 1% hypochlorite solution	15	3%	31	7%	3%	9	12%	5	7%	-5%
	Black containers present (discarded medicines, chemical waste)	390	82%	360	76%	-6%	53	72%	60	80%	8%
	Black containers have same colored plastic bags	93	20%	60	13%	-7%	16	22%	11	15%	-7%
	Black containers have 1% hypochlorite solution	122	26%	55	12%	-14%	21	28%	8	11%	-18%
Disposal of gloves	In red containers (correct)	298	63%	311	65%	3%	39	53%	49	65%	13%

Continued

		Level 2 health facilities with designated LABOR ROOMS					Level 3 health facilities with designated LABOR ROOMS				
		CFA 2017 (n=475)		CFA 2019 (n=476)		Change (% points)	CFA 2017 (n=74)		CFA 2019 (n=75)		Change (% points)
		n	%	n	%		n	%	n	%	
	In yellow containers (correct)	105	22%	104	22%	0%	24	32%	31	41%	9%
Disposal of dressing material	In red containers (correct)	152	32%	136	29%	-3%	22	30%	15	20%	-10%
	In yellow containers (correct)	233	49%	280	59%	10%	47	64%	54	72%	8%
Disposal of placenta	In yellow containers (correct)	414	87%	420	88%	1%	65	88%	72	96%	8%
Disposal of IV bottles and tubing	In red containers (correct)	328	69%	342	72%	3%	47	64%	60	80%	16%
	In black containers (acceptable)	77	16%	53	11%	-5%	10	14%	4	5%	-8%
Disposal of syringes	In white containers (correct)	12	3%	28	6%	3%	2	3%	9	12%	9%
	In red containers (wrong)	314	66%	287	60%	-6%	41	55%	47	63%	7%
Plastic waste cut into pieces before disposal	Syringes	197	41%	130	27%	-14%	35	47%	19	25%	-22%
	IV sets	171	36%	151	32%	-4%	31	42%	18	24%	-18%
	Catheters	133	28%	103	22%	-6%	23	31%	15	20%	-11%
	IV bottles	130	27%	116	24%	-3%	21	28%	14	19%	-10%

Table 2.8: Changes in laboratory service delivery: tests conducted in the last 30 days before CFA 2017 vs. CFA 2019

	Level 2 health facilities with designated Labs					Level 3 health facilities with designated Labs				
	CFA 2017 (n=450)		CFA 2019 (n=457)		Change (% points)	CFA 2017 (n=74)		CFA 2019 (n=74)		Change (% points)
	n	%	n	%		n	%	n	%	
Urine Pregnancy Test	222	49%	362	79%	30%	41	55%	62	84%	28%
Blood Grouping and RH typing	107	24%	190	42%	18%	29	39%	54	73%	34%
Hemoglobin(%)	138	31%	439	96%	65%	27	36%	73	99%	62%
Complete Blood Count (DC, TLC)	34	8%	267	58%	51%	35	47%	53	72%	24%
Glucose Tolerance Test	110	24%	148	32%	8%	31	42%	24	32%	-9%
Urine Sugar Test	217	48%	331	72%	24%	49	66%	58	78%	12%
Urine Albumin Test	207	46%	324	71%	25%	48	65%	57	77%	12%
Syphilis (VDRL/RPR)	137	30%	213	47%	16%	25	34%	35	47%	14%
Serum Urea and Creatinine	61	14%	111	24%	11%	31	42%	42	57%	15%
Tuberculosis	397	88%	no data			56	76%	no data		
Malaria	260	58%	392	86%	28%	37	50%	70	95%	45%
Kala-Azar	272	60%	291	64%	3%	43	58%	47	64%	5%
HIV	400	89%	437	96%	7%	57	77%	66	89%	12%
Hepatitis B (HBsAg)	80	18%	177	39%	21%	24	32%	49	66%	34%
Lab test reports provided to patients (printed or manually written reports)	177	39%	259	57%	17%	55	74%	55	74%	0%

Table 2.9: Changes in drug store management and use of web-based software (*e-Aushadhi*), CFA 2017 vs. CFA 2019

TABLE 2.9	Level 2 health facilities with designated drug storage rooms					Level 3 health facilities with designated drug storage rooms				
	CFA 2017 (n=469)		CFA 2019 (n=470)		Change (% points)	CFA 2017 (n=72)		CFA 2019 (n=74)		Change (% points)
	n	%	n	%		n	%	n	%	
Drug store in-charge ever received any training on use of e-Aushadhi web-based software	37	8%	130	28%	20%	20	28%	31	42%	14%
e-Aushadhi software being used in the facility	3	1%	193	41%	40%	4	6%	38	51%	46%
If YES, online indenting to District Drug Warehouse being done	2	67%	175	91%	24%	0	0%	32	84%	84%
if YES, drugs are also being issued against online indent to various departments within the facility	no data		56	29%		no data		9	24%	
Functional computer and printer dedicated for e-Aushadhi work is available in the facility	6	1%	133	28%	27%	5	7%	31	42%	35%
Drug store in-charge received training AND dedicated computer & printer available	1	0.2%	96	20%	20%	2	3%	24	32%	30%
Inventory management: only manual registers	no data		181	39%		no data		36	49%	
Inventory management: only software-based			45	10%				10	14%	
Inventory management: combined			131	28%				21	28%	
Data operator available for Drug Store			73	16%				22	30%	
NO mismatch in drug counts: as reported in e-Aushadhi software vs. physical verification										
Tablet Albendazole (400 mg) (Jar)	no data		17	4%		no data		3	4%	
Tablet Albendazole (400 mg) (Strip)			34	7%				9	12%	
Syrup Albendazole (200 mg/5ml) (Bottle)			28	6%				4	5%	
Tablet Zinc Sulphate dispersible (10 mg)			0	0%				2	3%	
Tablet Zinc Sulphate dispersible (20 mg)			35	7%				4	5%	
Tablet Iron folic acid – Large (Iron=100 mg + Folic acid = 500 mcg (0.5mg)			34	7%				12	16%	

Continued

	Level 2 health facilities with designated drug storage rooms					Level 3 health facilities with designated drug storage rooms				
	CFA 2017 (n=469)		CFA 2019 (n=470)		Change (% points)	CFA 2017 (n=72)		CFA 2019 (n=74)		Change (% points)
	n	%	n	%		n	%	n	%	
Tablet Iron folic acid – Small (Iron=20 mg + Folic acid =100 mcg (0.1mg)			6	1%				3	4%	
ORS 245 mmol/L for 12.5 gm Sachet			0	0%				0	0%	
ORS 245 mmol/L for 20.5 gm Sachet			35	7%				14	19%	
Tablet Iron folic acid – Blue Color (Iron=100 mg + Folic acid = 500 mcg (0.5 mg)			7	1%				1	1%	
Tablet Calcium + D3 (500 mg+250 IU/500 IU)			18	4%				4	5%	

2.3.2 Readiness score: facility-level and district-level summary changes over time

2.3.2.1 Facility-level summary changes from 2015-2019

Table 2.10 depicts the comparative summary statistics of the facility readiness score for 524 ID-matched delivery points across CFA 2015, 2017 and 2019.

Among the Level 2 facilities (n=455), both mean and median scores increased steadily over these 3 CFAs, though the mean increase was higher in the CFA 2017 vs. 2015 comparison (mean difference = 1.51, 95% confidence interval: 1.39, 1.63; p<0.0001) than the CFA 2019 vs. 2017 comparison (mean difference =0.18, 95% confidence interval: 0.07, 0.28; p=0.0011). Further, while the maximum score increased by only 0.45 points from 2015 to 2017 and did not change thereafter, the minimum score increased by 68% between 2015-2017 and by 34% between 2017-2019. Among the Level 3 facilities (n=69), both the mean and median scores increased from CFA 2015 to 2017 (mean difference = 1.39, 95% confidence interval: 1.1, 1.69; p<0.0001). However, the median score (7.5)remained static between CFA 2017 and 2019, while the mean increase (= 0.13, 95% confidence interval: -0.17, 0.44) was not a statistically significant change. In contrast to Level 2 facilities, both the minimum and maximum scores increased from 2015 to 2017, but decreased from 2017 to 2019 (though 2019 scores remained higher than the 2015 scores).

Figure 2.1 is the graphical representation of the above-described trend in the mean facility readiness scores for Level 2 and Level 3 delivery points over the 3 CFAs.

For Level 2 facilities, ANOVA was statistically significant (F-statistic = 324.14, p<0.0001), and the post-hoc Bonferroni multiple comparisons showed that there were statistically significant differences in mean facility readiness scores between CFA 2015-2017 (p<0.001), CFA 2015-2019 (p<0.001) and CFA 2017-2019 (p=0.047).

For Level 3 facilities, ANOVA was statistically significant (F-statistic = 43.81, p<0.0001), and the post-hoc Bonferroni multiple comparisons showed that there were statistically significant differences in mean facility readiness scores between CFA 2015-2017 (p<0.001) and CFA 2015-2019 (p<0.001), but not between CFA 2017-2019.

Table 2.11 categorizes Level 2 and Level 3 facilities according to the degree of change in facility readiness scores between CFA 2015-2017 and CFA 2017-2019. During the first (2015-2017) comparison period, 391 (86%) Level 2 facilities and 59 (86%) Level 3 facilities showed positive change, while 3% facilities at either level recorded zero change. In contrast, during the second (2017-2019) comparison period, 244 (54%) Level 2 facilities and 29 (42%) Level 3 facilities showed further positive change, while 6% Level 2 and 13% Level 3 facilities recorded zero change.

Table 2.10: Comparative summary statistics of facility readiness score – CFA 2015, 2017 and 2019

Type of Facility (n=524)		Facility Readiness Score			Mean difference (95% CI)	
		CFA 2015	CFA 2017	CFA 2019	CFA 2017 vs. CFA 2015	CFA 2019 vs. CFA 2017
Level 2 health facilities (n=455)	mean	4.99	6.5	6.68	1.51 (1.39, 1.63), **p<0.0001**	0.18 (0.07, 0.28), **p=0.0011**
	sd	1.23	1.04	1.01		
	median	5	6.59	6.82		
	min	0.93	1.56	2.09		
	max	8.41	8.86	8.86		
Level 3 health facilities (n=69)	mean	5.89	7.28	7.42	1.39 (1.1, 1.69), p<0.0001	0.13, (-0.17, 0.44), p=0.3798
	sd	0.98	1.25	0.94		
	median	5.91	7.5	7.5		
	min	3.18	4.42	3.95		
	max	8.41	9.32	9.09		

Note:524 id-matched facilities considered for paired t test analysis;
Mean difference = (2017 - 2015) & (2019 - 2017) scores
Legends: MNC: maternal and newborn care

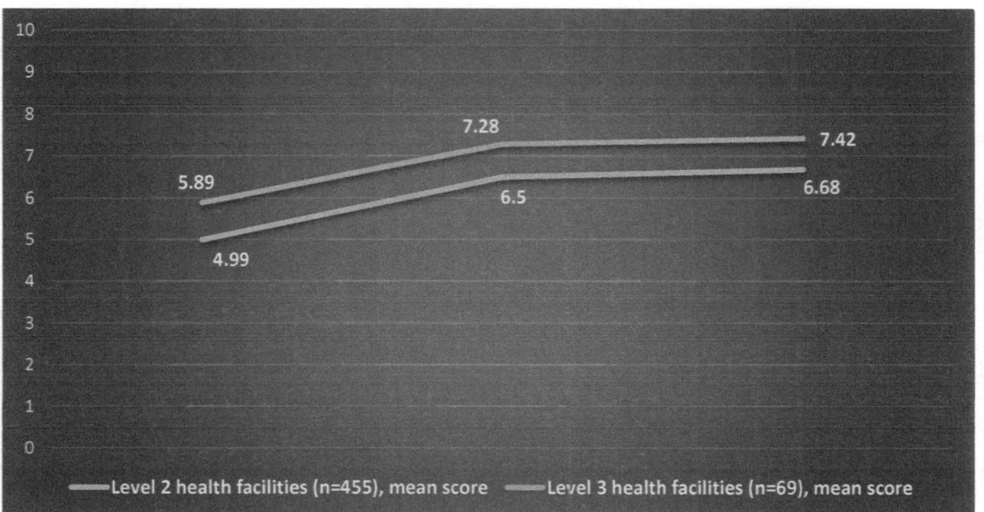

Figure 2.1: Trend of the mean facility readiness scores for Level 2 and Level 3 delivery points – CFA 2015, 2017 and 2019
Note: Level 2 facilities: p<0.0001 (ANOVA), significant differences between mean pairs CFA 2015-2017, CFA 2015-19 and CFA 2017-2019 (post-hoc Bonferroni multiple comparisons).Level 3 facilities: p<0.0001 (ANOVA), significant differences between mean pairs CFA 2015-2017 and CFA 2015-19, but not CFA 2017-2019 (post-hoc Bonferroni multiple comparisons).

Table 2.11: Facilities as per the degree of change in facility readiness scores

Level of change	CFA 2017 vs. CFA 2015				CFA 2019 vs. CFA 2017			
	Level 2 health facilities (n=455)		Level 3 health facilities (n=69)		Level 2 health facilities (n=455)		Level 3 health facilities (n=69)	
	n	%	n	%	n	%	n	%
negative change	52	11%	8	12%	183	40%	31	45%
no change (zero)	12	3%	2	3%	28	6%	9	13%
positive change, <3 points	330	73%	53	77%	240	53%	28	41%
positive change, ≥3 points	61	13%	6	9%	4	1%	1	1%

2.3.2.2 District-level summary changes from 2015-2019

Table 2.12 shows the district-level readiness scores for each of the 38 districts of Bihar across CFAs 2015, 2017 and 2019, and compares the mean change between CFA 2015 and 2017, as well as between CFA 2017 and 2019.

Between 2015 and 2017, all-but-one district (*Buxar*) showed increase in their readiness scores. In contrast, the scores decreased for 12 districts between 2017 and 2019. The overall mean score (for all districts of Bihar) increased from 5.22 during CFA 2015 to 6.62 during CFA 2017 (difference = 1.41, p<0.0001), and subsequently to 6.81 during CFA 2019 (difference from 2017 score = 0.19, p=0.07). Considering the scores from the 3 CFAs, 25 of the 38 districts in Bihar had demonstrated a continuous increase over the assessed time points. Among the remaining 13, all except *Buxar* (which recorded 0.03 decrease in score from CFA 2015 to 2017) had recorded a decline in their 2019 scores compared to 2017. However, for all these 13 districts, the readiness score during CFA 2019 remained higher than that during CFA 2015.

The 10 districts which were identified as high-priority ones under the national RMNCH+A program (highlighted in the table) demonstrated steady improvement of their scores over the 3 CFAs, except in the case of *Saharsa* district whose 2019 score decreased by 0.18 from the 2017 score, but remained higher than its 2015 score. The mean score for these 10 districts (*not shown in Table 2.12*) remained at par with the overall mean score for the state during each of CFA 2015 (mean score for high priority districts = 5.31 vs. state mean score = 5.22), CFA 2017 (6.58 vs. 6.62) and CFA 2019 (6.82 vs. 6.81).

Figure 2.2 is a heat map of the 38 districts of Bihar depicting the above-discussed district-level trends in readiness scores over time.

Table 2.12: Comparative summary statistics of district-level readiness scores – CFA 2015, 2017 and 2019

Districts	Common facilities (n=524)	CFA 2015 score	CFA 2017 score	CFA 2019 score	Score change: 2017 vs. 2015	Score change: 2019 vs. 2017	TREND
Araria	9	5.96	6.46	6.95	0.50	0.49	continuous increase
Arwal	6	5.11	6.59	6.93	1.48	0.34	continuous increase
Aurangabad	12	5.44	6.34	7.63	0.90	1.29	continuous increase
Banka	11	6.82	7.57	7.33	0.76	-0.25	decrease in 2019 from 2017, but score in 2019 >2015 score
Begusarai	17	4.48	6.16	7.16	1.68	0.99	continuous increase
Bhagalpur	16	5.94	7.57	7.13	1.62	-0.44	decrease in 2019 from 2017, but score in 2019 >2015 score
Bhojpur	16	4.38	6.18	6.71	1.80	0.54	continuous increase
Buxar	9	6.02	5.99	6.69	-0.03	0.70	decrease in 2017 from 2015, followed by increase in 2019 (score in 2019 > 2015 score)
Darbhanga	20	4.61	6.14	6.39	1.53	0.25	continuous increase
East Champaran	21	4.92	6.49	6.69	1.57	0.20	continuous increase
Gaya	24	6.02	6.95	7.22	0.93	0.27	continuous increase
Gopalganj	12	4.41	6.12	7.33	1.70	1.21	continuous increase
Jamui	10	5.20	6.74	6.96	1.53	0.22	continuous increase
Jehanabad	9	6.41	7.62	7.18	1.21	-0.44	decrease in 2019 from 2017, but score in 2019 >2015 score
Kaimur	10	5.48	7.61	6.64	2.14	-0.98	decrease in 2019 from 2017, but score in 2019 >2015 score
Katihar	14	5.20	6.69	6.69	1.48	0.003	continuous increase
Khagaria	7	5.78	6.76	6.01	0.98	-0.75	decrease in 2019 from 2017, but score in 2019 >2015 score
Kishanganj	9	5.45	6.92	7.47	1.46	0.55	continuous increase
Lakhisarai	6	6.63	7.00	7.68	0.37	0.68	continuous increase
Madhepura	14	5.26	7.65	6.69	2.39	-0.96	decrease in 2019 from 2017, but score in 2019 >2015 score
Madhubani	21	4.74	5.99	6.35	1.26	0.36	continuous increase
Munger	9	4.90	6.81	7.04	1.91	0.23	continuous increase

Continued

	Common facilities (n=524)	CFA 2015 score	CFA 2017 score	CFA 2019 score	Score change: 2017 vs. 2015	Score change: 2019 vs. 2017	TREND
Muzaffarpur	16	5.13	7.11	7.53	1.99	0.42	continuous increase
Nalanda	20	5.04	6.38	5.87	1.34	-0.51	decrease in 2019 from 2017, but score in 2019 >2015 score
Nawada	14	5.58	6.88	7.18	1.29	0.31	continuous increase
Patna	26	5.23	5.94	7.00	0.70	1.06	continuous increase
Purnia	9	5.49	6.72	6.73	1.23	0.01	continuous increase
Rohtas	19	4.28	6.21	7.03	1.93	0.83	continuous increase
Saharsa	10	6.25	7.27	7.09	1.02	-0.18	decrease in 2019 from 2017, but score in 2019 >2015 score
Samastipur	21	4.85	6.79	6.06	1.94	-0.73	decrease in 2019 from 2017, but score in 2019 >2015 score
Saran	20	3.91	6.57	6.23	2.66	-0.33	decrease in 2019 from 2017, but score in 2019 >2015 score
Sheikhpura	6	4.71	5.47	6.76	0.76	1.29	continuous increase
Sheohar	4	4.51	5.34	5.76	0.83	0.43	continuous increase
Sitamarhi	17	4.08	6.23	6.59	2.15	0.36	continuous increase
Siwan	17	4.26	6.98	6.15	2.73	-0.83	decrease in 2019 from 2017, but score in 2019 >2015 score
Supaul	11	5.50	6.43	6.79	0.94	0.36	continuous increase
Vaishali	16	5.16	6.84	7.09	1.68	0.25	continuous increase
West Champaran	16	5.07	6.15	5.94	1.08	-0.21	decrease in 2019 from 2017, but score in 2019 >2015 score
mean (sd) score		**5.22 (0.71)**	**6.62 (0.57)**	**6.81 (0.50)**			
mean difference (p-value)					**1.41 (p<0.0001)**	**0.19 (p=0.07)**	

Note: Highlighted districts represent the 10 high-priority districts identified under national RMNCH+A program

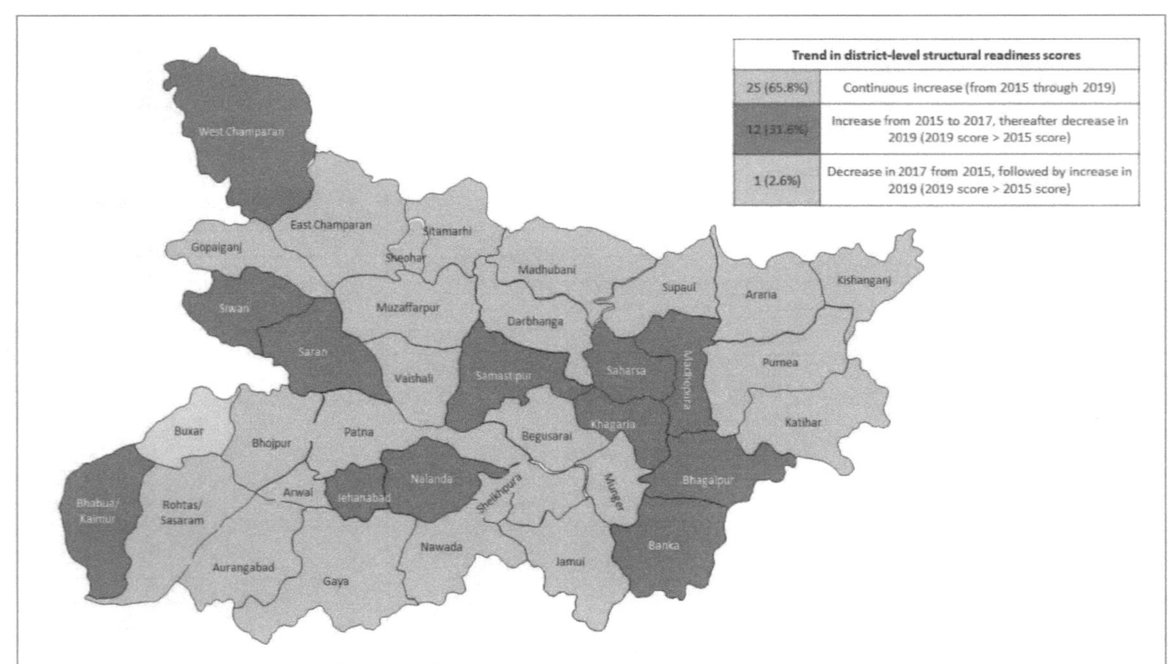

Figure 2.2: Heat map of the 38 districts of Bihar depicting district-level trends in facility readiness scores over time – CFA 2015, 2017 and 2019

2.4 Discussion

The formation of BTSP was based upon the premise that unless infrastructure, human resources, and supply chain needs within Bihar's public health system were identified and addressed, it would be an uphill challenge to achieve the desired RMNCH-focused program outcomes. Further, the achievements – if any, may not be sustainable in the long run unless such needs were addressed. In this context, the conceptualization and use of the CFAs as annual/ biennial exercises (by CARE India's Concurrent Measurement and Learning unit) was pivotal to generate, analyze and communicate ground-level evidence on structural readiness from the delivery points to the decision-making chambers. It was hoped that this process would enable the state health apparatus to use data in a timely manner to take action and progress towards data-based planning and monitoring of the health system strengthening effort.

The comparative analysis of data generated through CFA 2017 and 2019, especially when cross-referenced with relevant findings from CFA 2015 and 2016 (presented in the first paper of this book), identifies important trends related to the progress and shortcomings in achieving structural readiness of the public health facilities in Bihar. On one hand, the current analysis revealed remarkable progress in structurally preparing the facilities to deliver basic maternal and newborn care services – with improvements in related infrastructure, essential supplies, and supportive services like referral transport and laboratory facilities, as well as through recruitment of large number of ANM and GNM nurses. Yet, on the other hand, challenges were identified with bottlenecks in the supply chain system, and in recruiting and retaining specialist physician cadres. The following sections deliberate on the programmatic implications of these findings, and further examine if the overall progress had been in-sync with the priorities laid down under the national RMNCH+A program. Based on these considerations, the paper attempts to present a candid assessment of the diagonal health system strengthening program in Bihar, and propose future directions.

2.4.1 The success: structurally preparing facilities to deliver basic maternal and newborn care services

The results from across different domains of the facility-level health system strengthening effort – infrastructure, supplies, human resources, referral transport systems, and laboratory services – clearly indicated that the BTSP had a constant focus on structurally preparing the health facilities to deliver basic maternal and newborn care services.

Since CFA 2015, there had been steady progress in relocating/ creating NBCCs inside the labor rooms – the proportion of such facilities increased from 55% (any facility type) in 2015 to 76% in 2017 and 82% in 2019 for Level 2 facilities, and to 89% in 2017 and 88% in 2019 for Level 3 facilities. Simultaneously, the availability of functional equipment related to newborn care (like baby weighing machines, radiant warmers, and AMBU bags with neonatal oxygen masks) increased from CFA 2015 to 2017, and further improved by CFA 2019. The availability of essential medicines like Oxytocin, Misoprostol, magnesium sulphate, antibiotics, antihypertensives and vitamin K injections remained stable and/or improved during CFA 2019, compared to 2017. Additionally, the supply of reproductive health/ family planning commodities like condoms, IUCD-375, sanitary napkins, iron and folic acid tablets, oral and emergency contraceptive pills increased across all facilities. These structural changes were supported by remarkable improvements in two related services areas – increased availability of emergency transport, and improved service provision by the laboratories. Finally, the facility-level capacity to deliver basic maternal and newborn care services was greatly boosted by the appointment of large number of ANM and GNM nurses – considering both regular and contractual recruitments.

By CFA 2019, more than 4600 ANM nurses were available for service at Level 2 facilities and nearly 400 at Level 3 facilities; while over 300 GNM nurses were available for service at Level 2 facilities and over 1700 at Level 3 facilities – all notable increases from CFA 2017. While the ANMs typically performed the bulk of outreach activities (especially pertaining to reproductive health, family planning, maternal and childhood nutrition, and wellbeing), both ANM and GNM nurses were capable of providing at least BEmONC services. Indeed, the BTSP had been conducting a nurse mentoring program (AMANAT) since 2014 which was specifically geared to develop BEmONC service competency among the nurses at Level 2 facilities, and CEmONC service competency at Level 3 facilities.[32, 43, 67] The focus on increased recruitment of the nursing cadre was indeed a pragmatic step to counter the lack of physicians at both levels of health facilities, at least for BEmONC service provision.

These results certainly reflect a purposeful effort by the BTSP to address system-wide parameters that would improve the structural capacity of public health facilities to deliver basic maternal and newborn care services. While acknowledging that there are more areas which need to be strengthened to achieve the desired facility-level capability, the current approach certainly seems to be in the right direction.

The impact of focused interventions by local governments and their development partners to improve maternal and/or newborn care services in public health facilities has been widely studied in low- and middle-income country (LMIC) settings. A 2015 national survey of health facilities in Nepal[90] demonstrated that most public health facilities had availability of basic equipment and essential medicines to provide maternal and newborn care – a result of dedicated government-level efforts over two decades. Basic equipment like thermometers, fetoscopes, blood pressure apparatus, baby weighing machines, and AMBU bags with neonatal oxygen

119

masks were available in at least 80% public hospitals. Medicines like injectable uterotonics were present in all hospitals and in 90% of primary health centers, while injectable antibiotics were present in 83% of hospitals and 55% of primary health centers. Tomlin et. al.[91] surveyed public health facilities in Ethiopia, India (*Uttar Pradesh* state) and Nigeria (*Gombe* State) in 2012 and 2015 to study the impact of ongoing RMNCH programs. They collected data on human resources availability, infrastructure and essential supplies, and used this data to measure the readiness of facilities to perform 4 signal functions[92] – management of labor using the partograph, active management of the third stage of labor using prophylactic uterotonics, general infection prevention, and newborn-specific infection prevention (clean cord care). The proportion of facilities that were deemed to be prepared to deliver good quality maternal and newborn care services (i.e. performing all 4 signal functions) increased from 22% (2012) to 35% (2015) in Ethiopia, and from 2% to 23% in *Uttar Pradesh*, India. In both cases, the overall improvement was facilitated by increased supply of equipment and consumables to perform management of labor and clean cord care, as well as the increased availability of uterotonic drugs, partographs and urine testing kits. In contrast, the proportion of facilities performing all 4 signal functions decreased from 17% in 2012 to none in 2015 in *Gombe*, Nigeria – a consequence of a breakdown in the supply chain for most essential commodities, lack of clean running water, and absence of skilled birth attendants.

These findings not only support the BTSP's focused approach, but also underline the fact that in absence of basic infrastructure, drugs, equipment, and human resources, efforts to improve the quality of care may have little or no impact. This observation was further corroborated by Vesel et al.[93], who examined the facility-level factors affecting essential newborn care service delivery in rural Ghana. They found that the peripheral secondary and primary-level clinics in Ghana

suffered from stock-out of essential commodities like neonatal bags and masks (not available in
37% of clinics), suction apparatus (25% clinics), antibiotics like Ampicillin (60% clinics), and
Dexamethasone (stock-out in all clinics). Further, 90% of these facilities suffered from absence
of a stable power supply or back-up power supply. These serious infrastructure shortcomings,
coupled with the fact that only 31% of the health workforce were trained in caring for the sick
newborn, translated to only one-third of all babies being born in a facility which could provide
life-saving basic neonatal resuscitation.

Hence, while the actual impact of BTSP's initiatives may only be assessed through future data on
service utilization and health outcomes, it can certainly be said that these persistent and
purposeful efforts shall go a long way to improve the facility-level readiness to deliver maternal
and newborn care services.

2.4.2 The concerns: challenges in meeting infrastructure, supply chain and human resources
needs

While the achievements outlined above indicated commendable progress in some areas, the
analysis also revealed a number of other areas requiring further attention including upgrading/
maintaining physical infrastructure, recruiting and/or retaining physician cadres, and addressing
complexities in supply chain management.

2.4.2.1 Infrastructure and human resources

About one-third of all facilities exhibited some signs of infrastructural damage during both
CFAs, and over three-fourths of facilities at either level did not have an adequate number of
labor tables as per RMNCH+A program specifications. Some basic amenities like a fully
equipped handwashing station (elbow tap with running water and soap) remained unavailable in
almost half of the labor rooms at Level 2 facilities, in 60% of the designated maternity wards,

and in almost all the laboratories during CFA 2019. However, such lack of basic conveniences in public health facilities was certainly not unique to Bihar – a WHO/ UNICEF survey[94] of more than 66,000 health facilities across 54 LMICs had found that 38% of all facilities did not have supply of clean water, 35% lacked water and soap for handwashing, while 19% had compromised sanitation systems. The situation was found to be particularly worrying in the primary health centers, where these deficiencies posed a great threat towards infection prevention while conducting deliveries or providing basic newborn care.

In the human resources domain, the BTSP faced continuing challenges in recruiting and/or retaining physicians in the public health facilities, especially with regards to specialist physician cadres – a finding common to all CFAs since 2015. Not more than 20% of the sanctioned strength of OBGYNs, pediatricians, anesthesiologists or general surgeons were available for service in Level 2 facilities during CFA 2019. The situation was marginally better at Level 3 facilities. In the first paper of this book, it has been noted that the absence of specialist physicians was a common finding in most states in India, and this crisis disproportionately affected the public health systems. In poorer states like *Uttar Pradesh* as well as better-off ones likes *Andhra Pradesh* and *Telangana*, between 20-30% of the required strength of OBGYNs, pediatricians, anesthesiologists or surgeons were found to be present at any level of public health facilities.[81, 82]

A survey of 24 hospitals and 60 health centers in Malawi[95] – a country that has long invested in improving maternal and newborn care services – found that while most facilities had adequate supplies of essential equipment, medicines and consumables, notable shortcomings existed in addressing human resource requirements. About 12% of the surveyed hospitals and health facilities did not have any clinically trained health care provider (physician or others) assigned to maternity care. Further, none of the available clinical service providers in more than 40%

hospitals and 75% health centers were trained in BEmONC. Indeed, the absence of physicians,

or sometimes even any skilled providers to conduct deliveries, has been widely reported from

surveys of public health facilities in LMICs like Bangladesh, Nepal, Haiti, Malawi, Senegal, and

Tanzania.[96, 97]

2.4.2.2 Supply chain

The challenges were more complex with the supply chain system. While supplies related to

maternal and newborn care services had notably improved by CFA 2019, there were persistent

challenges in improving availability of basic equipment like stethoscopes, blood pressure

instruments and oxygen cylinders, or available stock of essential drugs like Salbutamol,

Labetalol and Methyldopa in labor rooms. Deterioration was also observed with the availability

of normal saline and Ringer's lactate solutions, as well as for common consumables like cotton

and gauze rolls, and intravenous cannulas and syringes. Thus, the supply chain system presented

inconsistencies compared to the overall analysis. In this context, the data on utilization of the *e-

Aushadhi* software platform for inventory management by the facility drug storage rooms

provides some insights into the possible fault lines. During CFA 2019, over 80% of facilities

using *e-Aushadhi* at either level utilized this software to indent drugs from the district drug

warehouses. However, less than 30% of these facilities routinely allocated drugs through *e-

Aushadhi* across the different departments within a facility, like the labor rooms and maternity

wards. The inconsistent use of *e-Aushadhi* introduced the risk of inaccurate interpretation of the

reported stock-in (or stock-out) status of supplies in the electronic system – which might also

have remained out-of-sync with the true availability status in the labor rooms and maternity

wards for some facilities. In fact, during CFA 2019, a mismatch was observed between the physical count of select drugs and the data in *e-Aushadhi* at over 90% of Level 2 and 80% of Level 3 facilities. It becomes evident that data regarding the indenting process must get accurately reflected in the *e-Aushadhi* system in real-time, to demonstrate actual status of supplies within the facility at any given point of time to ensure accurate commodity management.

Similar challenges in strengthening the pharmaceutical supply chain capability (for medicines and consumables) emerged from an assessment of 499 health facilities in Ethiopia in 2014 and 2015. Since 2009, the Ethiopian government, with support from the UNFPA, systematically invested to ensure the availability of medicines and supplies related to reproductive health at all public health facilities. The surveys revealed disparities in stock-in status between primary care centers and the higher-level facilities – for e.g., stock-in of 7 essential reproductive health medicines was reported by only 20% primary care facilities in contrast to 86% tertiary care facilities. Delays in replenishing stocks was a major roadblock to ensuring availability of essential supplies in over 30% of primary care facilities, and this was found to be due to inefficiencies in correctly requesting re-supplies. Additional delays within the supply chain system (purchase and distribution) further deteriorated the situation. However, year-on-year improvements were noted in managing stocks at the facility level through timely reporting of accurate data.[98] Identical challenges were also reported from a 2017 WHO SARA (service availability and readiness assessment) survey of 60 randomly selected primary health centers in Enugu State, Nigeria – which had implemented decentralized district-level health system reforms to strengthen its primary health care system since 2005. On average, only 46 of the 100 listed equipment and 27 of the 102 essential drugs were available in the clinics on the day of the assessment. The supply chain was found to be particularly weak for drugs and consumables related to communicable diseases and maternal health.[99] Bintabara et. al[100] surveyed 905 health facilities in Tanzania, and found that 70% of these were incapable of providing BEmONC services due to chronic non-availability of equipment and supplies – suction machines, vacuum aspirators, sterilization machines and examination lights were not available in 75-90% of the facilities, while more than 50% of facilities reported stock-outs of IV fluids, magnesium sulphate and antibiotics for both mother and newborn.

While the data from Bihar does not necessarily point towards supply-related disparities between Level 2 and Level 3 facilities, the state may do well to recognize the importance of training all drug store managers in using *e-Aushadhi* to both procure and distribute the supplies – as that would address a root-cause of supply chain problems. Notably, 80% of the state-level funds for infrastructure development and supply chain management goes to the Bihar Medical Services & Infrastructure Corporation Limited[64] for centralized procurement and distribution, while the remaining 20% funds are given directly to facilities to allow local purchases to meet emergency stock-outs of essential supplies. Updating and ensuring accurate facility level data will improve efficiency. Hence, the correct use of e-Aushadhi, and the extension of electronic procurement/ management platforms for equipment and consumables as well, can be a key step to unwinding the supply chain gridlocks.

2.4.3 Contextualizing progress: BTSP approach and the national RMNCH+A program priorities

The BTSP, like the national RMNCH+A program, was fundamentally based on the idea that a health system strengthening approach towards improving RMNCH program outcomes (i.e. a diagonal approach) was necessary to overcome longstanding bottlenecks across the system and achieve sustainable progress. In doing so, the national program urged states to prioritize functionalizing public health facilities which served the most underdeveloped districts.

Concurrently, it emphasized the need to preferentially develop the lowest level of facilities that could provide RMNCH care, arrange for emergency referral transport systems in the rural and remote areas, and recruit health workforce cadres that would work closest to the communities.[60, 85] These priorities identified under the national program were grounded in evidence. Powell-Jackson et. al[101] assessed the structural quality of primary health centers in India based on data from the 2007-08 national District Level Household and Facility Survey, and found statistically significant variations not only between the different states, but also between the rural and urban areas within a district. The gap was particularly high for availability of essential medicines (18-point difference) and equipment (10-point difference), as well as with regards to basic clinic infrastructure (15-point difference). They concluded that most primary health centers failed to meet the minimum structural standards set by the Government of India, and noted this as an important reason for even the poor, rural population opting for costlier private health care services.

For the BTSP, aligning with the national program priorities meant focusing on strengthening the Level 2 facilities, and the 10 high priority districts identified under RMNCH+A. The analysis of the facility readiness scores provided an assessment of this alignment. 86% of Level 2 facilities demonstrated improvement in their individual scores between 2015 and 2017, while 54% further improved between 2017 and 2019. Overall, both the mean and median scores for Level 2 facilities improved steadily and significantly between 2015, 2017 and 2019. Further, the minimum score more than doubled from 2015 to 2019, indicating that the weakest facilities benefitted the most from BTSP's interventions. However, there remained significant variation in MNC structural readiness within the Level 2 facilities, as the maximum score from CFA 2019 was four times the minimum – though this disparity had reduced from the nine-fold difference in

2015. In contrast, progress was much less pronounced at Level 3 facilities, though these facilities

(district and sub-divisional hospitals) are typically better equipped and staffed compared to the

Level 2 facilities – as evidenced by their higher mean and median scores at any time point. These

findings certainly point towards a conscious choice made to address the weaker structural

conditions of the Level 2 facilities as a priority measure.

At the district-level, 9 out of the 10 high priority districts demonstrated continuous improvement

of their scores over the 3 time-points. Only 1district showed a decline in score from 2017 to

2019, though the latter remained higher than its 2015 score. More significantly, the mean score

for these 10 districts remained at par with the overall mean score for the state (considering all 38

districts) during each of CFA 2015, 2017 and 2019.

In addition to the above findings, it is also worth recollecting that the BTSP had achieved

remarkable progress in increasing the availability of functional ambulances and ensuring more

emergency referral transportations at both Level 2 and Level 3 facilities. It had also supported

the government to ensure that ANM and GNM nurses were increasingly recruited (through

regular or contractual modes) and made available at all facilities to ensure at least BEmONC

service delivery. The nursing staff represent a category of health care providers that remains

closest to the communities, especially at the Level 2 facilities. Thus, in more than one way, the

BTSP's focus to structurally prepare public health facilities to deliver basic maternal and

newborn care services was likely to benefit all, but more so the rural and remote communities.

2.4.4 Overall assessment and future directions

The critical analysis of BTSP's successes and shortcomings in structurally strengthening Bihar's

public health facilities demonstrated that achieving an overall statewide progress for the universe

of health facilities within a resource-poor healthcare system can be painfully slow, and this progress is often inconsistent. In particular, while the rate of improvement was much steeper from CFA 2015 to 2017, it proved to be extremely challenging to hold on to this pace of change over the subsequent 2 years (CFA 2017 to 2019). This was evidenced by analysis of readiness scores at the facility-level as well as at the district-level.

Evidence from consecutive facility-level assessments (WHO SARA surveys) in Ethiopia in 2016 and 2018[102] substantiate the fact that achieving consistent improvement in the availability of basic necessities like infrastructure, equipment and medicines remains extremely challenging and is a remarkably slow process. While the proportion of Ethiopian facilities with available ambulances increased from 67% in 2016 to 84% in 2018, only about 60% of facilities had 4 out of the 6 basic equipment (as listed in SARA) during either survey. Among the 24 essential medicines enumerated, only ORS, Amoxicillin and zinc were available in more than 50% of the surveyed facilities, while a meagre 28% of these facilities reported availability of all medicines. Overall, 4% of BEmONC-level facilities and 1% of CEmONC-level facilities satisfied the criteria for service readiness.

While the facility-level assessments from Bihar as well as other LMIC settings broadly convey a common theme – that a health system strengthening approach to achieve program outcomes might often require more time to show results, it remains important to appreciate the complexity of the process. Abdalla et. al[103] conducted an in-depth analysis of the trends in RMNCH and nutritional program indicators in Bihar between 2012 and 2017. They found that while there were sharp gains made during 2012 and 2013, the trends were varied thereafter. It is also worth remembering that between 2011 and 2013, CARE India was implementing facility-based and outreach-based solutions focusing on these indicators in 8 programmatically prioritized districts under the Integrated Family Health Initiative program.[18] In contrast, after the BTSP was launched in November 2013, CARE India was relegated to a technical and managerial supportive

role, with the state government taking ownership of implementing interventions. The results

from this study were hence reflective of the fundamental difference in service delivery

approaches between a development partner and a government, which was likely attributable to

the differences in organizational culture.[104] However, the researchers also emphasized that

adopting a health system strengthening approach towards RMNCH outcomes (as was the case

under BTSP) would necessarily mean a slower progress to achieving desired outcomes, as the

path traverses through the challenging terrains of improving infrastructure, addressing supply

chain complexities, and recruiting skilled human resources for health. Hence, in all fairness, the

Bihar government should be accorded more time to fully integrate all interventions within its

own system, and premature conclusions on the lack of rapid improvements may be unjust. It had

previously been observed that prolonged periods of intensive program implementation directly

by external partners can actually do more harm than good to a local public health system – as the

latter has no incentive to own the development process and improve from within.[105]

The BTSP recognized this reality, and had been supporting the Bihar government towards these

long-term goals. Data from CFA 2019 demonstrated that a large number of data entry operators

(considering regular and contractual appointments) had been recruited and made available at

both Level 2 and Level 3 health facilities – a step that would support the process of generating

and managing facility-level data as part of the regular operations. Further, there had been notable

recruitments of program management staff like block-level health managers, community

mobilizers, monitoring and evaluation officers, account managers and district health managers –

representing a workforce that shall facilitate improved ground-level implementation of BTSP's

interventions. In the long run, these determined steps support creating a pathway for sustainability, as the onus is gradually shifted from the development partners to the state health system.

2.4.5 Limitations

The current paper relied on analysis of existing operational research data that was concurrently generated through the CFAs conducted by CARE India's Concurrent Measurement and Learning unit in 2017 and 2019. The CFAs were mandated to generate detailed facility-level data to track changes in infrastructure, supplies and human resources that happened as a result of BTSP's interventions. Consequently, the objectives of the current paper were bound by the goals of the CFAs, and did not permit answering further research questions like assessing the change in service utilization, if any. However, this is a common limitation of working with field-level data which has its own objective of being gathered for the purposes of monitoring and evaluating progress, and is not exclusively collected for research purposes.

Second, the facility-level assessments in Bihar did not use a globally standardized instrument like the 2015 WHO SARA tool (or its earlier versions) that had been widely used to assess health facilities as part of evaluating health system strengthening efforts in LMICs.[106] While the WHO SARA tool and the CFA instrument share commonalities across the data collection domains, the latter was fundamentally based on national guidelines and tools developed by the Government of India.[39, 40] Further, the CFA data collection instrument continuously evolved since its first application during the 2015 CFA, and its expansion had matched the incremental interventions initiated under BTSP. By 2017, the CFA instrument was exhaustive enough to collect data on every functional aspect of a public health facility in Bihar, ranging from labor room infrastructure to the use of inventory management software in drug storage rooms. Thus, the purpose of the CFA tool was not to provide data to construct population-based indicators or allow cross-national comparisons (like the WHO SARA tool), but to be specific to the needs of the BTSP – to help measure the ground-level needs in public health facilities of Bihar, and track progress over the course of time.

Finally, the facility readiness score was not constructed following standard statistical procedures that would otherwise be warranted to create a complex, nuanced index reflecting the overall facility level service delivery scenario by using high level indicators. Indeed, the current facility readiness score was developed as an operational score to provide a summary understanding of the progress of facility-level interventions. The selection of 44 parameters to construct this score was done on the basis of repeated consultations between stakeholders who represented the state officials and the development partners. A similar process was followed by researchers who monitored the equitable progress of primary healthcare reforms in *Kerala* state.[107, 108] They recognized that it was often necessary to tailor indicators based on operational realities like relevance to the ongoing program and data availability from the facilities being monitored. The team created an initial list of 812 primary health care indicators based on global and national frameworks, but subsequently curtailed the same to 23 locally relevant ones through a modified Delphi process involving key stakeholders like policymakers, public health experts, primary care providers and front-line workers. The development of the summary score for BTSP followed a similar process, and its scope remains limited to understanding the program in Bihar. This operational score shall be expanded in future to measure the progress in service areas beyond maternal and newborn care.

2.5 Conclusion

The BTSP's efforts to improve the structural readiness of public health facilities in Bihar is indeed a work in progress. There have been notable successes, especially with regards to equipping the facilities to deliver basic maternal and newborn care services, while some shortcomings exist. Based on these considerations, the paper proposes a few measures to support and accelerate progress.

Developing and/or maintaining facility-level infrastructure – particularly basic amenities like functional handwashing stations (with running water and soap), adequate labor tables, and appropriate sanitation systems – is indispensable for ensuring proper service provision. The CFA data had clearly identified the facilities suffering from these infrastructural gaps, and the BTSP should prioritize addressing these areas by setting specific goals for the blocks and districts. If targeted funding is channeled through the Bihar Medical Services & Infrastructure Corporation Limited, the remedial measures can be quickly implemented.

In contrast, the chronic shortage of specialist physicians is a much more complicated issue to address. One way to address this problem might be through adopting the "task shifting" approach[109] which has been widely applied in HIV programs to address the crisis of specialized manpower. Task shifting involves a rational redistribution of tasks from highly qualified health workers to others in the workforce through tailor-made training programs. Consequently, such an approach not only enables a health system to maximally use its available human resources, there is also ample evidence that quality of care can be ensured and indeed improved through this process.[110] The BTSP demonstrated similar innovation by staffing the facilities with nursing cadres to ensure that at least basic maternal and newborn care provision was not affected due to non-availability of physicians. In the same spirit, the BTSP may consider training the available nursing and physician cadres to meet specific facility-level requirements for strengthening CEmONC service delivery capacity, which would otherwise require a number of specialist positions.

Third, it remains important for the BTSP to keep working towards addressing the myriad complexities within Bihar's supply chain system. In particular, it is pivotal that the BTSP targets equipping all facilities with electronic/ web-based systems for managing the inventory, and simultaneously trains the designated personnel to use such systems correctly and efficiently. The analysis demonstrated that erroneous stock-in (or stock-out) status of the supplies in the electronic system would potentially compromise the procurement and distribution at the facility and district levels.

Finally, the current analysis and discussion highlights the importance of government ownership of the diagonal health system strengthening program in Bihar, while the development partners transition to a technical support role. Even if this approach may result in delays in achieving desired RMNCH outcomes, the paper unambiguously endorses this process as the right path forward. It is encouraging to note that while the BTSP was initially funded for a four-year period (2014-2017), the support is being currently sustained to ensure continuity of the system-wide efforts and to develop system-driven mechanisms that would ensure sustainability of the interventions within Bihar's public health system.

Chapter 3: Is the structural readiness of public health facilities to provide maternal and newborn care services associated with facility performance? Findings from the 2018-2019 facility-level assessments in Bihar, India

3.1 Introduction

The Government of Bihar, one of the most resource-poor and densely populated states in India, has collaborated with the Gates Foundation since 2010 to strengthen the capacity of its public health system to deliver reproductive, maternal, newborn and child health (RMNCH) and nutritional services. Between 2011 and 2013, the Integrated Family Health Initiative (IFHI) – with CARE India as an implementation partner – sought to accelerate progress in these areas through facility-based and outreach-based solutions in 8 programmatically prioritized districts of the state.[18] Based on experiences gained during the IFHI period, it soon became necessary to re-imagine this partnership to address the foundational needs within Bihar's public health system – specifically, those pertaining to infrastructure, supply chain and human resources that potentially affected both the quantity and quality of facility-level RMNCH service delivery. The statewide Bihar Technical Support Program (BTSP) was hence initiated in November 2013 to provide a comprehensive structure to the technical support by development partners (like CARE India) to the state government to strengthen Bihar's public health system, while keeping the focus on RMNCH outcomes. The interventions were scaled up to cover all 38 districts of the state.[27, 28] The BTSP developed a novel structure of health governance whereby state-, district- and block-level technical support teams were created and fully embedded within the state health system. This was necessary to co-develop health system interventions with the state government, and transfer ownership of the implementation and monitoring activities. To support these efforts, CARE India formed a functionally independent Concurrent Monitoring and Learning (CML) Unit to oversee establishment and management of data systems that could generate evidence and transfer it from facilities to the policymaking levels. The details regarding the genesis and governance structure of BTSP has been discussed in the first paper of this book. At the facility-level, the BTSP adopted a two-pronged strategy. On one hand, BTSP utilized annual/ biennial comprehensive facility assessments (CFAs) conducted by the CML Unit to identify and address gaps in facility-level infrastructure and essential supplies, as well as rationalize the distribution of available health workforce. It was hoped that this approach would help to improve the "facility readiness" (or, structural readiness) of public health facilities to deliver RMNCH services. Simultaneously, the BTSP also conducted an on-site nurse mentoring programs to develop competency among the general nurse midwives (GNM nurses) and auxiliary nurse midwives (ANM nurses) in providing basic and comprehensive emergency obstetric and newborn care (BEmONC/ CEmONC) services. This intervention was known as the AMANAT program – an acronym for *Apaatkalin Matryitwa evam Nawjat Tatparta,* which means emergency obstetric and newborn care (EmONC) service readiness.[22]AMANAT was targeted to improve the quality of care, and consequently, the "facility performance". **Figure 3.1** depicts the simplified conceptual framework to understand the facility-level interventions to strengthen facility readiness and facility performance to improve RMNCH outcomes.

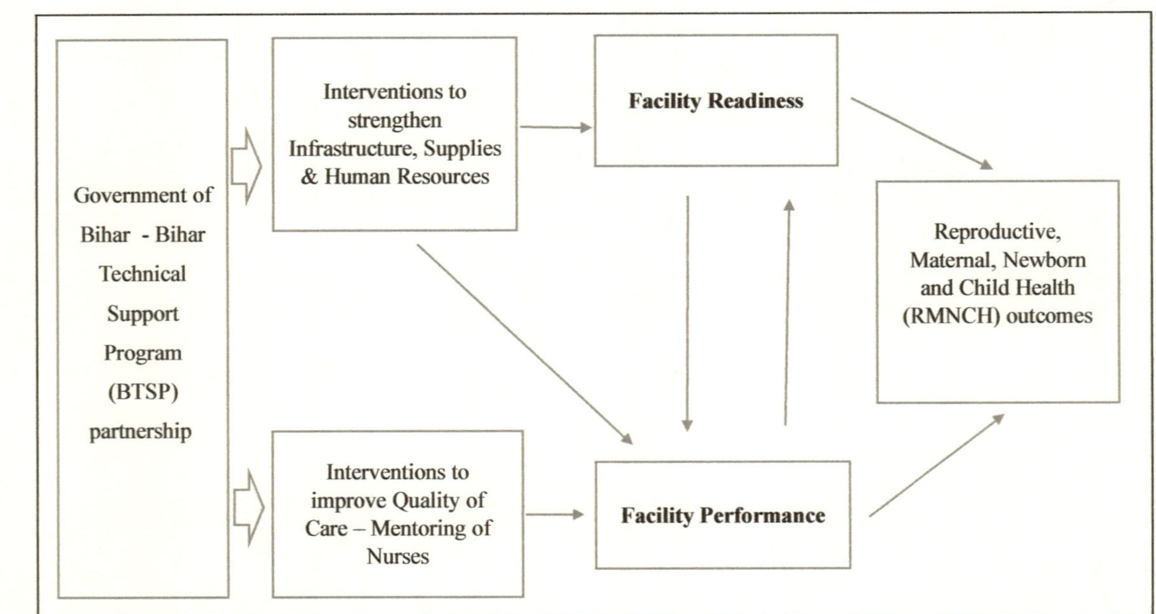

Figure 3.1: Government of Bihar – Bihar Technical Support Program (BTSP) partnership to strengthen Facility Readiness and Facility Performance to improve Reproductive, Maternal, Newborn and Child Health (RMNCH) outcomes

3.1.1 Progress in facility readiness: findings from the CFAs (2015-2019)

Between 2015 and 2019, the CML Unit of CARE India had conducted 4 CFAs to collect

exhaustive data on the condition of physical infrastructure, availability of functional equipment,

consumables and essential drugs in all Level 2 (primary health centers, community health centers

and referral hospitals) and Level 3 (sub-divisional hospitals and district hospitals) facilities

across Bihar which conducted deliveries – and the findings had been presented in previous

manuscripts. The detailed analysis from CFA data has been presented in the first two papers of

this book. The analysis demonstrated that structurally strengthening Bihar's public health

facilities was challenging, and the results were mixed. By 2019, almost all facilities provided

24x7 delivery services in their labor rooms and had designated newborn care corners which are

earmarked areas to provide immediate post-delivery care to the newborns. The most consistent

improvement (2015–2019) noted was the availability of functional equipment, medicines and

consumables related to conducting deliveries and providing essential newborn care (i.e., in the

labor rooms). These structural changes were supported by improvements in availability of

emergency transport (ambulances), and service provision by the laboratories. Further, by CFA

2019, the facility-level capacity to deliver basic maternal and newborn care services was greatly

boosted by the appointment of a large number of auxiliary and general nurse midwives through

both regular and contractual (i.e. hired under different projects as term-limited employees)

recruitment channels. These improvements were captured in the facility readiness scores.

Interestingly, while the score had increased sharply between CFA 2015 and 2017 across both

Level 2 and Level 3 health facilities, the rate of increase declined between CFA 2017 and 2019.

Continuing lack of some basic infrastructural amenities (like handwashing stations, labor tables), supply chain gridlocks stemming from inefficient facility-level inventory management, and the difficulty in recruiting and retaining physicians likely contributed to this slowed progress.

3.1.2 A brief history of the AMANAT interventions

CARE India's nurse-mentoring initiative was first started in 2012 as part of the IFHI program. Between 2012 and 2014, the "mobile nurse mentoring and training program"[57, 58] was conducted across 80 public health facilities across the 8 programmatically prioritized districts of Bihar to develop competency among nurses posted in the labor rooms. Under this initiative, a team of 2 expert nurses, hired from renowned organizations in India, was assigned to 4 selected health facilities to provide mentorship to (mostly) the ANM nurses. Each mentor team conducted 1 week-long training at each assigned facility, completing 4 facilities in a month – and this cycle was repeated about 6 times. The mentorship involved skill-building through hands-on training and supervised patient-care sessions.

After the launch of BTSP, this mobile nurse mentoring initiative evolved into the AMANAT *Buniyadi* (meaning "basic" training to develop competency in providing BEmONC services at Level 2 health facilities) and AMANAT *Vyapak* (meaning "comprehensive" training to develop competency in providing CEmONC services at Level 3 health facilities) programs.[68-70]Between 2015 and 2017, on-site mentoring was conducted for both GNM and ANM nurses in 4 phases, involving 80 high-volume facilities per phase. A pair of expert mentor nurses (contracted from different reputed institutions in India) were assigned to 4 health facilities to conduct on-site mentoring and training within the labor rooms – spending 1 week per facility, and covering all 4 facilities within 1 month. The mentors would return to each assigned facility for similar week-long trainings and observation of practices for a total of 7-9 consecutive months. The training involved intensive exercises in skill-building through gaining correct knowledge (basic procedures and infection prevention, documentation, reporting), actively participating in simulation-based group training sessions, as well as conducting supervised deliveries and identifying and addressing the complications that arose.

In 2018, it was decided to further modify AMANAT to ensure that the program could be sustained through utilizing the instilled capacity (through AMANAT) within Bihar's public health system to train unskilled providers, as well as to ensure continuous training of AMANAT-trained providers. This revised edition was called AMANAT *Jyoti*. About 10-20 AMANAT-trained government nurses with demonstrated professional efficiency were screened and selected as AMANAT mentors from across the public health facilities within each district, and brought together as part of a "district mentoring team". Each such team was a recognized entity within the state health system. The specific roles included conducting induction training for fresh appointee nurses as well as strengthening EmONC-specific training in the nursing schools. At the facility-level, a pair of AMANAT mentors – called nurse mentoring supervisors – were designated to conduct BEmONC and CEmONC training, following the existing schedule (described above). Thus, the AMANAT *Jyoti* program envisioned developing a strong, sustainable system for continuous mentoring and training of nurse providers to ensure a standard quality of care in BEmONC and CEmONC service delivery.

3.1.3 Progress in facility performance: findings from AMANAT assessments (2015-2017)

A number of publications had discussed findings from the BTSP's nurse mentoring initiative. Ghosh et. al[68] analyzed data from the direct observation of more than 55,000 deliveries across 320 health facilities covered by the AMANAT intervention between 2015 and 2017. They identified notable improvements in the providers' ability to correctly identify complications like postpartum hemorrhage and birth asphyxia between the first and final weeks of mentoring. Based on data from 240 AMANAT facilities over the same time period, Creanga et. al[22] found that the intervention contributed to significant increase in knowledge (by 30%) and well as infection control (31%), intrapartum (29%) and newborn care (24%) practices among the mentored nurses, after controlling for potential confounders like the type of facility, delivery volume, presence of equipment etc. Indeed, multiple studies had identified the positive impact of AMANAT interventions in enabling mentee nurses to ask more relevant questions on past medical history, post-partum hemorrhage and intrapartum asphyxia, and better provide evidence-based management of these complications.[68, 69, 111] The overall quality of care with respect to labor room practices (delivery and essential newborn care) was found to be significantly improved in the AMANAT facilities compared to their non-mentored counterparts. However, the proportion of essential tasks completed was quite low in the mentored facilities even after 3 months of training (44% vs. 30% in non-mentored facilities), and it further reduced (to 39%) at the 1-year follow-up assessment. Hence, even with AMANAT mentoring, less than half of the recommended steps in managing labor and the newborn were being complied with.[70] Similarly, an evaluation of facility-level neonatal resuscitation simulation training (conducted under AMANAT) revealed that while 31% more facilities administered effective positive pressure ventilation and 13% more correctly assessed infant heart rate after the training, these gains declined by at least 20% over the next year.[112] These findings highlighted the success of the AMANAT intervention in improving provider knowledge and practices, but equally underlined the need to continue this mentoring as a periodic intervention to ensure sustainability of the gains – a realization that shaped the AMANAT *Jyoti* program in 2018.

3.1.4 Objective

There is no doubt that the BTSP's dual interventions to improve facility readiness (structural

readiness) as well as build competency among the nursing cadre remain key steps to address the

foundational weaknesses within Bihar's public health system. The trends in facility readiness

(based on CFA data) had been analyzed and presented in the first two papers of this book.

However, it remained important to understand if facility readiness was positively and

significantly associated with facility performance, since that would provide evidence of

synergistic progress, as envisioned under BTSP.

The current paper has 2 objectives. The first objective is to determine whether the facility-level

performance changed, and this is accomplished by comparing the baseline (May-December,

2018) and endline (October-December, 2019) assessment data from the AMANAT *Jyoti*

program. The second objective is to assess the association between facility readiness and endline

facility performance in providing maternal and newborn care (MNC) services. This is

accomplished by analyzing data from facility-level assessments (CFA and AMANAT *Jyoti*)

conducted in 2018 and 2019 by the CML Unit of CARE India.

3.2 Methods

In order to address the study objectives, a secondary analysis of quantitative data generated

through two separate assessments conducted by CARE India's CML Unit – the 2019 CFA and

the 2018-2019 assessment of the AMANAT *Jyoti* program was conducted. More specifically,

two operational scores were used – the facility-level MNC structural readiness score (*henceforth*

referred to as facility readiness score) and the facility-level MNC performance score (*henceforth*

referred to as facility performance score) to test the association between facility readiness and

performance. The sections below describe the data sources and the operational scores in details.

141

3.2.1 CFA 2019 and the facility readiness score

The detailed methodology of the 2019 CFA as well as the development of the facility readiness

score has been described in details in the second paper of this book. Since the current paper

utilizes the facility readiness score, a brief description is presented below.

The 2019 CFA was a cross-sectional assessment of all public health facilities in Bihar which

conducted a minimum of 100 deliveries in the preceding year. These facilities were either Level

2 or Level 3 health facilities in the state, as the Level 1 facilities (village-level health sub-

centers) mostly do not conduct deliveries. CFA 2019 was conducted in August-September 2019

and covered 552 facilities. Data was collected on the availability of human resources, the

condition (infrastructure/ equipment/ drugs/ consumables) of labor rooms, maternity wards, drug

storage rooms and laboratories, as well as the referral transport services and bio-medical waste

management/ infection control practices.

Based on operational considerations, a limited number of parameters were selected from the

CFA data which reflected human resources, infrastructure and essential supplies related to

delivering MNC services at the health facilities. The selection process involved a series of

iterative consultations between all stakeholders in the BTSP – state-level policymakers, select

group of district and block-level health care providers, CARE India leadership, and public health

experts. **Panel 3.1** depicts the list of 44 parameters that were selected to develop the facility

readiness score. These parameters were also reflective of the service-specific structural readiness

for management of normal deliveries and emergency management of postpartum hemorrhage,

newborn care including management of birth asphyxia, and infection prevention.

In order to calculate the facility readiness score, each parameter in Panel 3.1 was awarded a score

of 1 for its presence and 0 for absence (opposite scoring for negatively-framed questions) – so that a higher score represented better structural readiness. If data was not collected for a

particular parameter at a facility, it was awarded 0 points. Thus, the possible score range for each

facility was 0-44. The actual score for each facility was next transformed to a 0-10 scale using

the formula: $transformed\ (final)\ score = \left(\left(\frac{10-0}{44-0}\right) * (X - 44)\right) + 10$, where X is the

original facility readiness score.

Panel 3.1: Indicators used to develop the Facility Readiness Score

Sl. No.	Indicators	Domains	Service-specific readiness		
			Management of normal deliveries and emergency management of PPH	Newborn care (including management of asphyxia)	Infection prevention
1	At least one ANM or GNM Nurse available for service	Human Resources	x	x	x
2	At least one Pediatrician available for service			x	x
3	At least one OBGYN available for service		x	x	x
4	At least one General Duty Medical Officer/ Internal Medicine Physician available for service		x	x	x
5	All walls in LR have at least 6 feet tiles	Infrastructure	x	x	x
6	No sign of water seepage from wall or roof in LR		x	x	x
7	Facility has a new born care corner inside the LR			x	
8	No area with diameter 1 feet or more in the LR roof where plaster is chipped-off		x	x	x
9	At least 1 invertor/generator (power back-up) available in LR		x	x	
10	Elbow tap available in LR		x	x	x
	Availability of at least one functional:	Supplies - Equipment			
11	digital/manual baby weighing machine in LR			x	
12	radiant warmer in LR			x	
13	BP apparatus (digital/mercury) in Facility		x		
14	stethoscope in Facility		x		
15	Fetal Doppler/Fetoscope in Facility		x	x	
16	Haemoglobinometer in Facility		x		
17	Pulse oximeter in Facility		x		
18	Phototherapy machine in LR			x	
19	Suction machine (Electric / Foot Operated) in LR			x	

Continued

Sl. No.	Indicators	Domains	Service-specific readiness		
			Management of normal deliveries and emergency management of PPH	Newborn care (including management of asphyxia)	Infection prevention
20	AMBU Bag (250 ml or 500 ml) in LR			x	
21	Mask size 0 or 1 in LR			x	
22	Needle Cutter /Burner in Facility		x	x	x
23	Electric Sterilizer OR Boiler OR Autoclave Machine in Facility		x	x	x
24	Yellow color coded container in LR		x	x	x
25	Red color coded container in LR		x	x	x
26	White color coded container in LR		x	x	x
	Availability of at least one:				
27	Cap in LR		x	x	x
28	Apron in LR		x	x	x
29	Face Mask in LR	Supplies - Consumables	x	x	x
30	Chromic Catgut – No. 1 with round body needle in LR		x		
31	Gauze rolls (any size) in Facility		x	x	
32	Sanitary Pad (disposable) in Facility		x		
33	Intravenous Cannula 16G/18G/20G/22G/24G in Facility		x		
34	Foley's catheter (16) in Facility		x		
35	Mucus Sucker (Dee Lee's Type) in LR			x	
36	Cord clamp in LR			x	

Continued

Sl. No.	Indicators	Domains	Service-specific readiness		
			Management of normal deliveries and emergency management of PPH	Newborn care (including management of asphyxia)	Infection prevention
	Availability of any stock-in quantity of:				
37	ANY uterotonic in the LR (oxytocin, misoprostol, methyldopa)	Supplies - Drugs	x		
38	Gel Lignocaine (2% or 5%), Injection Lignocaine/ Lidocaine (2% or 5% vial) in Facility		x		
39	Povidone Iodine (5% Betadine) Solution in Facility		x		x
40	Ringer Lactate (500 ml/ 1000 ml) in Facility		x		
41	20 IU Oxytocin in Facility**		x		
42	Injection Magnesium Sulphate (500 mg/ml ampoule) in Facility		x		
43	Availability of ANY hypertensive: Injection Labetalol (any strength), Capsule Nifedipine (5 mg) in Facility		x		
44	Availability of ANY Antibiotic in any strength: Capsule Amoxicillin, Injection Amoxicillin, Capsule Ampicillin, Injection Ampicillin, Injection Ceftriaxone, Inj. Amikacin, Injection Gentamycin in Facility		x	x	

Note: Positive Indicators were scored as 1 for 'yes' and 0 for 'no'; Negative Indicators were scored as 0 for 'yes' and 1 for 'no'.

Legends: ANM: auxiliary nurse midwives; GNM: general nurse midwives; OBGYN: Obstetrician & Gynecologist; LR: Labor Room; PPH: postpartum hemorrhage

**Availability of at least 20 IU Oxytocin in the facility was separately awarded a score (in addition to "presence of any uterotonics") since this is the minimum loading dose required to start treatment for PPH.

3.2.2 The 2018-2019 assessment of AMANAT *Jyoti*

In 2018, when the AMANAT *Jyoti* program was targeted to be implemented in over 350 Level 2

and Level 3 health facilities across Bihar, the CML Unit had planned pre- and post-intervention

assessments. Accordingly, the baseline data was collected from May-August, 2018 in facilities

where BEmONC training was scheduled (henceforth referred to as BEmONC facilities), and

from September-December, 2018 in facilities where CEmONC training was scheduled

(CEmONC facilities). The endline data collection took place between October and December

2019 at both BEmONC and CEmONC facilities. It is worth noting here that ideally, all Level 2

facilities in Bihar are expected to provide at least BEmONC services, while all Level 3 facilities

are expected to provide CEmONC services. However, in reality, not all Level 2 facilities in Bihar

can perform the 7 WHO BEmONC signal functions.[38] On the other hand, among the Level 3

facilities, some sub-divisional hospitals can only provide BEmONC services while blood banks

(a key CEmONC signal function) are not present in most facilities.

As of December 2020, baseline data was available from 158 health facilities, while endline data

was available from 134 among these health facilities. Operational delays in recruiting and

training the expert nurses, as well as in implementing the assessments over several phases led to

this lag in the availability of complete pre- and post-intervention data from the facilities. Further,

the stringent procedures for data quality check and cross-verification from the facilities delayed

availability of some additional data.

The baseline and endline assessments were cross-sectional in design. The nurse mentoring

supervisors conducted both baseline and endline assessments using a previously validated

checklist[63] to ascertain compliance with the expected standards for delivery and newborn care

practices. The data collection tool was expansive, and required information on the clinical condition of the pregnant women prior to being admitted, the mode of transport to arrive at the facility, pre-delivery complications (like antepartum haemorrhage, hypertensive disorders, malpresentation, multiple pregnancy, cord prolapse etc.) and their management in the facility. These data were collected through client interviews and checking the records in the facility. However, the core part of the assessment comprised of directly observing the practices pertaining to conducting normal vaginal deliveries, managing postpartum haemorrhage, providing essential newborn care including management of birth asphyxia, as well as adhering to basic infection prevention practices. Direct observation of provider practices while delivering care is often considered as the gold standard in identifying the strengths and shortcomings of the process.[63, 113] The baseline assessment was conducted during the first week of AMANAT *Jyoti* training at a health facility. Thus, the baseline assessment was not a pre-training exercise. As part of the assessment, the nurse mentoring supervisors were required to directly observe the conduct of at least 1 normal delivery with provision of essential newborn care over the 1 week period at a given facility. It was understood that direct observation of management of complications like postpartum haemorrhage and birth asphyxia would vary depending on the patient requirements. The idea was to ensure direct observation of at least 1 delivery and 1 newborn care per facility, with or without complications management. However, in practice, multiple deliveries were observed in most facilities, courtesy of the high patient volume. All observations were made during the regular training hours (between 9 am – 5 pm). This baseline assessment took place between May-December, 2018. The endline assessment was conducted following a similar protocol, at least 9 months after the baseline assessment (October-December, 2019).

The data was collected electronically through hand-held android tablets (tablet-sized personal computer devices) using a hybrid custom-built platform enabled with inherent logic checks developed in-house, bridging between proprietary licensed Survey-CTO platform[87] and the Open

Data Kit (free and open-source software) platform[88] – a process followed during the 2019 CFA.

To ensure the quality of the data being collected (in addition to the built-in logic checks

described above), trained data quality monitoring coordinators from the CML Unit routinely

cross-checked the data and resolved any inconsistencies after consulting with the nurse

mentoring supervisors.

3.2.3 Development of the facility performance score

The current paper was restricted to the analysis of non-identifiable program data collected

through direct observation of deliveries (normal vaginal deliveries with management of

postpartum haemorrhage if needed), newborn care (including management of birth asphyxia if

needed), and infection prevention practices in the assessed health facilities. While detailed data

was collected through the direct observations, it was decided to focus on selecting a limited

number of parameters that would reflect these core practices targeted through AMANAT *Jyoti*,

and would be in-sync with the facility readiness score described above. The process of selecting

such parameters was also identical to the one followed during development of the facility

readiness score, as described in the second paper of this book. **Panel 3.2** depicts the 45

parameters that were selected through iterative consultations between implementation team

(policymakers at the state level along with a select group of district and block-level health care

providers) and the technical support team (CARE India leadership ground team and public health

experts).

These 45 parameters were next used to develop the facility performance score – an operational

score reflective of the core training imparted through the AMANAT *Jyoti* program. As depicted

in the Panel, all outcomes were recorded as binary – i.e., a yes or no response to specific standards of care being followed during the observations. Each parameter was accorded equal weightage – 1 point for complying with the standard of care, and 0 otherwise. Negatively-framed responses were reverse-coded, so that a higher score would reflect a better level of facility performance. If more than 1 delivery was observed at a particular facility, the average of the scores for each parameter was awarded. Thus, the possible score range for each facility was 0-45. However, the scoring system also recognized that several of these parameters depended on the clinical requirements of the patient. For example, episiotomy was not routinely required in all deliveries, and hence the 3 related parameters (episiotomy done if indicated, sterile scissors used, and repair sutured) were scored only if it was appropriate. In cases where episiotomy was not required, these parameters were neither included in calculating the numerator (total score) or the denominator (maximum possible score). A similar method was followed for scoring on the management of postpartum hemorrhage (5 parameters) and management of birth asphyxia (3 parameters). So, for example, in a situation where the patient needed episiotomy but did not suffer from postpartum hemorrhage, and the newborn needed bag-and-mask ventilation, the maximum score was 40.

The actual score for each facility was next transformed to a 0-10 scale using the formula:

$$transformed\ (final)\ score = \left(\left(\frac{10-0}{Max.Score-0}\right) * (Y - Max.Score)\right) + 10,$$ where Y is the original facility performance score and the maximum score is dependent on the specific clinical requirements of the mother and the newborn.

Panel 3.2: Indicators used to develop the Facility Performance Score

Domains	Sl. No.	Indicators
Management of normal deliveries and emergency management of PPH	1	Temperature measured before delivery
	2	Pulse measured before delivery
	3	Blood pressure measured before delivery
	4	Abdominal examination before delivery
	5	Fetal heart rate measured before delivery
	6	Vaginal examination before delivery
	7	Oxytocin was not given before delivery *(scored 0 if given before delivery)*
	8	Fundal pressure was not applied anytime during labor *(scored 0 if applied)*
	9	All the instruments used were sterile or disinfected
	10	Among the episiotomy done, how many were indicated
	11	Sterile scissors were used for episiotomy (among all episiotomy)
	12	Episiotomy/tear repaired
	13	Administration of oxytocin for active management of the third stage of labor
	14	Counter cord traction given
	15	Uterine massage done
	16	Placental lobes and membranes checked for completeness
	17	Genital tract exploration performed after delivery
	18	Vaginal packing not done *(scored 0 if done)*
	19	Use of sanitary pad for perineal support
	20	Mother transferred from labor room to the ward after delivery
	21	At least one IV line (catheter) established in the PPH patient
	22	Administration of at least 20 IU Oxytocin for PPH management
	23	IV fluid Started
	24	Blood pressure measured at least once post delivery
	25	Pulse measured at least once post delivery

Continued

Domains	Sl. No.	Indicators
Essential newborn care (including management of asphyxia)	26	Baby wiped dry
	27	Eyes wiped with sterile wet gauze
	28	Baby covered in a cloth separate from drying cloth
	29	Cord checked for pulsations before clamping
	30	Delayed umbilical cord clamping (1 minute after birth) done
	31	Sterile material (thread) used to tie the cord
	32	Sterile blade / scissors used to cut cord
	33	Nothing was applied to cord stump *(scored 0 if applied)*
	34	Skin to skin contact initiated within 5 minutes of birth
	35	Breastfeeding initiated within 1 hour of delivery
	36	Birth of baby registered in birth/ delivery register
	37	Weight of the baby taken
	38	Suction/Stimulation done (if required)
	39	Bag-mask ventilation done after suctioning or stimulation (if required)
	40	Baby stable and managed in the same facility
Infection prevention practices	41	Delivery attendant(s) wore aprons
	42	Delivery attendant(s) wore masks
	43	Delivery attendant(s) wore caps (cover hair)
	44	Delivery attendant(s) washed hands with soap and water
	45	Delivery attendant(s) wore gloves

Note: Positive Indicators were scored as 1 for 'yes' and 0 for 'no'; Negative Indicators were scored as 0 for 'yes' and 1 for 'no' - noted in the Panel.
Highlighted indicators are complications/ procedures which may vary as per patient needs:
#10-12: Episiotomy; #21-25: PPH; #38-40:Birth asphyxia
Legends: PPH: postpartum hemorrhage; IV: intravenous

3.2.4 Data analysis

As mentioned earlier, the current paper utilized data that was available with the CML Unit of CARE India as of December 2020. Though the baseline AMANAT *Jyoti* assessment data was available from 158 health facilities, the endline data was available for 134 among them. Thus, the analysis utilized the 134 health facilities which had both baseline and endline data from the AMANAT *Jyoti* assessments. The facility ID – which remained constant for a facility across the different assessments – was used to create a common dataset containing the facility readiness score (from CFA 2019) and facility performance scores (from AMANAT *Jyoti* baseline and endline assessments) for each facility. Data on the monthly facility-level delivery volume for 2019 was available for all facilities covered during CFA 2019, and the same was used to calculate the average monthly delivery volume for 2019.

The data was analyzed using STATA SE v.15.[41] The raw data was first tabulated as the number of directly observed deliveries (N) at the 134 public health facilities, the number of observed correct practices (n), and the proportion (n/N). This analysis was done for each of the 45 parameters depicted in Panel 3.2 – separately for baseline and endline – and the change in percentage-points was noted. Subsequent analysis focused on conducting paired t tests for the mean change in facility performance scores (endline vs. baseline), as per the type (BEmONC/ CEmONC) and level (Level 2/ Level 3) of facility. A two-sided p-value <0.05 was considered to be significant. The mean facility readiness score and the mean delivery volume as per facility level and facility type were also analyzed.

The main focus of the analysis was to test the association between facility performance and facility readiness. The facility performance score from the endline assessment of AMANAT *Jyoti* (conducted in October-December 2019) was the dependent outcome variable, and the facility readiness score from CFA 2019 (conducted August-September 2019) was the key independent variable of interest. It was decided to test this association while controlling for the baseline facility performance score (based on baseline AMANAT *Jyoti* assessment, May-December 2018), the type (BEmONC/ CEmONC) or level (Level 2/ Level 3) of facilities, and the average facility-level monthly delivery volume for 2019. Multiple linear regression (ordinary least squares method) modeling was done with the endline facility performance score as a continuous outcome. Additionally, multiple multinomial logistic regression modeling was done using tertiles of the endline facility performance score (lowest/ middle/ highest tertiles) as category boundaries.

3.2.5 Ethical approval

The use of CFA and AMANAT *Jyoti* assessment data in this manuscript was determined as "not human subjects research" (under 45 CFR 46) by the Institutional Review Board at Columbia University, New York, USA (Protocol #IRB-AAAT1461, decision dated July 20, 2020). The data generated through the CFAs related to select facility-level characteristics like availability of human resources, physical condition of the health facilities in terms of infrastructure, functionality of equipment and supply of drugs and consumables. The data from assessment of the AMANAT *Jyoti* program related to select obstetric and newborn care practice indicators. This data was completely de-identified by CARE India at source, and the data used for purposes of this analysis did not have any identifiers to be traced back to any individual respondent. Thus, all data used in this paper were retrospective and secondary, and also did not contain any individual-level identifiers (non-human subject data).

3.3 Results

134 public health facilities had both baseline and endline AMANAT *Jyoti* assessment data and were included in the analysis. 121 of these were Level 2 facilities (all provided BEmONC services), while the remaining 13 belonged to Level 3 (9 provided CEmONC services while 4 provided BEmONC services). Thus, 125 were BEmONC facilities and 9 were CEmONC. As discussed under the methods section, while all Level 2 facilities were BEmONC facilities (despite not satisfying all 7 signal functions), only some Level 3 facilities – not all – could provide CEmONC-level services (except presence of blood bank). Among these facilities, 132 were covered during CFA 2019 which had an inclusion criterion of a minimum 100 deliveries in the preceding year for each facility.

3.3.1 Descriptive overview of facility-level performance

Table 3.1 shows the detailed information from the direct observation of deliveries at the 134 facilities, and subsequent analysis of the proportion of correct practices for each of the 45 assessment parameters. A total of 1039 deliveries were observed during the baseline AMANAT *Jyoti* assessment, and 468 during the endline assessment. However, the total number of observations varied for each parameter, and has been shown in the table. A decline in performance was observed for 9 (20%) of the 45 parameters between baseline and endline. Administering oxytocin for active management of the third stage of labor, performing neonatal resuscitation in babies with birth asphyxia, and subsequently stabilizing and managing these babies in the same health facility declined by 14-17 percentage-points; while repairing the episiotomy incisions or vaginal tears, as well as the practice of transferring mothers from labor rooms to the wards after delivery decreased by 7-9 percentage-points.

During the endline assessment, there were 16 (36%) parameters which had a score of less than 50% – meaning that the nurse providers mostly performed wrong actions for these steps. Measuring temperature and pulse and conducting abdominal examination before delivery were routinely ignored in over 90% of observations (despite improvement from the baseline assessment). In over 60% of the observations at endline, pre-delivery maternal blood pressure was not measured and oxytocin was not injected during the third stage of labor. The eyes of the newborn were not wiped with a sterile gauze in over 80% of instances. Three among the 5 observed infection prevention practices recorded poor compliance during the endline assessment –delivery attendants wore facial masks during 33% and caps during 14% of the observations, while they washed hands with soap and water before conducting deliveries in only 21% of instances.

Assessment of the parameters dependent on the patients' clinical requirements – episiotomy, management of postpartum hemorrhage, and birth asphyxia showed varied results. While 179 episiotomies were done at baseline, only 6 (3%) were judged to have been clinically indicated – this proportion improved to 27% at endline (10 out of 37), but still remained very concerning. The proportion of episiotomy incisions and/or vaginal tears which were repaired decreased from 35% (299/865) at baseline to 26% (110/423) at endline. Sanitary pads were used to provide perineal support during delivery in less than 70% of the observations at endline. The proportion of correct practices followed in managing postpartum hemorrhage improved between the 2 assessments – in over 80% of the observations during endline, 20 IU oxytocin was administered as a loading dose (20 percentage-points improvement) and intravenous fluids were started (4 percentage-points improvement). However, measurement of blood pressure after delivery was observed on 43% occasions, while measurement of pulse was observed on 21% occasions during both assessments. With regards to the management of birth asphyxia, while simulation/suction

was done in 72% of the necessary cases during endline (a decline as noted earlier), bag-and-mask

ventilation was performed in 87% of the required instances, representing a 13 percentage-points

improvement of this life-saving practice.

Table 3.1: Indicators used to develop the facility performance score (data from assessment of AMANAT *Jyoti*)

Domains	Sl. No.	Indicators	Baseline (May-December, 2018)			Endline (October-December, 2019)			Change (%points)
			N	n	%	N	n	%	
Management of normal deliveries and emergency management of PPH	1	Temperature measured before delivery	1039	9	0.9%	468	7	1.5%	0.6%
	2	Pulse measured before delivery	1039	69	6.6%	468	40	8.5%	1.9%
	3	Blood pressure measured before delivery	1039	277	26.7%	468	165	35.3%	8.6%
	4	Abdominal examination before delivery	1039	15	1.4%	468	33	7.1%	5.6%
	5	Fetal heart rate measured before delivery	1039	381	36.7%	468	217	46.4%	9.7%
	6	Vaginal examination before delivery	990	774	78.2%	455	410	90.1%	11.9%
	7	Oxytocin was not given before delivery *(scored 0 if given before delivery)*	858	807	94.1%	418	403	96.4%	2.4%
	8	Fundal pressure was not applied anytime during labor *(scored 0 if applied)*	865	663	76.6%	423	380	89.8%	13.2%
	9	All the instruments used were sterile or disinfected	710	134	18.9%	333	199	59.8%	40.9%
	10	Among the episiotomy done, how many were indicated	179	6	3.4%	37	10	27.0%	23.7%
	11	Sterile scissors were used for episiotomy (among all episiotomy)	179	36	20.1%	37	24	64.9%	44.8%
	12	Episiotomy/tear was repaired	865	299	34.6%	423	110	26.0%	-8.6%
	13	Administration of oxytocin for active management of the third stage of labor	704	356	50.6%	392	145	37.0%	-13.6%
	14	Counter cord traction given	789	447	56.7%	410	337	82.2%	25.5%
	15	Uterine massage done	794	406	51.1%	412	362	87.9%	36.7%
	16	Placental lobes and membranes checked for completeness	791	229	29.0%	409	214	52.3%	23.4%
	17	Genital tract exploration performed after delivery	814	747	91.8%	415	371	89.4%	-2.4%
	18	Vaginal packing not done *(scored 0 if done)*	830	781	94.1%	414	395	95.4%	1.3%
	19	Use of sanitary pad for perineal support	817	121	14.8%	404	107	26.5%	11.7%
	20	Mother transferred from labor room to the ward after delivery	802	698	87.0%	399	318	79.7%	-7.3%

Continued

Domains	Sl. No.	Indicators	Directly observed deliveries at 134 public health facilities						Change (%points)
			Baseline (May-December, 2018)			Endline (October-December, 2019)			
			N	n	%	N	n	%	
Management of normal deliveries and emergency management of PPH	21	At least one IV line (catheter) established in the PPH patient	112	98	87.5%	37	33	89.2%	1.7%
	22	Administration of at least 20 IU Oxytocin for PPH management	112	68	60.7%	37	30	81.1%	20.4%
	23	IV fluid Started	112	92	82.1%	37	32	86.5%	4.3%
	24	Blood pressure measured at least once post delivery	112	48	42.9%	37	16	43.2%	0.4%
	25	Pulse measured at least once post delivery	112	24	21.4%	37	8	21.6%	0.2%
Essential Newborn care (including management of asphyxia)	26	Baby wiped dry	850	461	54.2%	420	279	66.4%	12.2%
	27	Eyes wiped with sterile wet gauze	785	34	4.3%	390	76	19.5%	15.2%
	28	Baby covered in a cloth separate from drying cloth	850	459	54.0%	420	273	65.0%	11.0%
	29	Cord checked for pulsations before clamping	850	273	32.1%	420	280	66.7%	34.5%
	30	Delayed umbilical cord clamping (1 minute after birth) done	672	413	61.5%	362	262	72.4%	10.9%
	31	Sterile material (thread) used to tie the cord	672	513	76.3%	362	275	76.0%	-0.4%
	32	Sterile blade / scissors used to cut cord	672	200	29.8%	362	251	69.3%	39.6%
	33	Nothing was applied to cord stump *(scored 0 if applied)*	779	778	99.9%	388	388	100.0%	0.1%
	34	Skin to skin contact initiated within 5 minutes of birth	126	97	77.0%	171	128	74.9%	-2.1%
	35	Breastfeeding initiated within 1 hour of delivery	785	453	57.7%	390	242	62.1%	4.3%
	36	Birth of baby registered in birth/ delivery register	850	811	95.4%	420	410	97.6%	2.2%
	37	Weight of the baby taken	849	812	95.6%	423	410	96.9%	1.3%

Continued

Domains	Sl. No.	Indicators	Directly observed deliveries at 134 public health facilities						Change (%points)
			Baseline (May-December, 2018)			Endline (October-December, 2019)			
			N	n	%	N	n	%	
	38	Suction/Stimulation done (if required)	174	152	87.4%	58	42	72.4%	-14.9%
	39	Bag-mask ventilation done after suctioning or stimulation (if required)	102	76	74.5%	31	27	87.1%	12.6%
	40	Baby stable and managed in the same facility	174	113	64.9%	58	28	48.3%	-16.7%
Infection prevention practices	41	Delivery attendant(s) wore aprons	865	656	75.8%	423	319	75.4%	-0.4%
	42	Delivery attendant(s) wore masks	865	160	18.5%	423	140	33.1%	14.6%
	43	Delivery attendant(s) wore caps (cover hair)	865	51	5.9%	423	61	14.4%	8.5%
	44	Delivery attendant(s) washed hands with soap and water	867	103	11.9%	423	90	21.3%	9.4%
	45	Delivery attendant(s) wore gloves	865	850	98.3%	423	416	98.3%	0.1%

Note: Positive Indicators were scored as 1 for 'yes' and 0 for 'no'; Negative Indicators were scored as 0 for 'yes' and 1 for 'no' - noted in the Panel.
Highlighted indicators are complications/ procedures which may vary as per patient needs:
#10-12: Episiotomy; #21-25: PPH; #38-40:Birth asphyxia
Legends: PPH: postpartum hemorrhage; IV: intravenous

3.3.2 Summary analysis of the scores

Table 3.2 presents the summary analysis of facility performance (n=134) and facility readiness (n=132) scores. The mean facility performance score increased significantly from baseline to endline among both levels and both types of facilities – but the increase was higher among Level 3 (1.56, p=0.0005, n=13) and CEmONC (1.82, p=0.0029, n=9) facilities, than among Level 2 (0.32, p =0.0288, n=121) and BEmONC (0.33, p=0.0168, n=125) facilities. In contrast, the mean facility performance scores were mostly higher at both baseline and endline for Level 2 vs. Level 3 facilities (baseline: 5.81 vs. 4.26; endline: 6.13 vs. 5.82) and BEmONC vs. CEmONC facilities (baseline: 5.76 vs. 4.28; endline: 6.09 vs. 6.10).

The mean facility readiness score was typically higher among Level 3 (8.11) and CEmONC (8.26) facilities, than among Level 2 (6.78) and BEmONC (6.81) facilities. The mean monthly delivery volume for 2019 was 226 for Level 2 and 232 for BEmONC facilities, while it was much higher – 657 for Level 3, and 761 for CEmONC facilities.

Table 3.2: Summary analysis of the scores

		Facility Level		Facility Type	
		Level 2 health facilities	Level 3 health facilities	BEmONC health facilities	CEmONC health facilities
Facility performance score (AMANAT *Jyoti*)	#Facilities (n=134)	121	13	125	9
	Baseline (mean (sd))	5.81 (1.33)	4.26 (0.91)	5.76 (1.35)	4.28 (0.84)
	Endline (mean (sd))	6.13 (1.05)	5.82 (1.09)	6.09 (1.05)	6.10 (1.18)
	Mean difference (95% CI)	0.32 (0.03, 0.60)	1.56 (0.84, 2.28)	0.33 (0.06, 0.61)	1.82 (0.83, 2.81)
	p-value	0.0288	0.0005	0.0168	0.0029
Facility readiness score (CFA 2019)	#Facilities (n=132)	119	13	123	9
	Mean (sd)	6.78 (0.92)	8.11 (0.79)	6.81 (0.94)	8.26 (0.65)
	Median	6.82	8.18	6.82	8.64
Delivery volume (2019)*	#Facilities (n=132)	119	13	123	9
	Mean (sd)	225.85 (109.11)	657.10 (372.79)	232.31 (118.28)	760.49 (388.22)
	Median	204.92	563.75	207.58	592.5

*Reflects the monthly facility-level delivery volume for 2019, based on CFA 2019 data.

Legends: MNC: maternal & newborn care; BEmONC: basic emergency obstetric and newborn care; CEmONC: comprehensive emergency obstetric and newborn care; SD: standard deviation; CI: confidence interval

3.3.3 Testing the association between facility readiness and performance scores

Tables 3.3 and **3.4** demonstrate results from the regression analyses with endline facility performance score as the dependent outcome variable and facility readiness score as the key independent variable of interest. 132 facilities had both facility performance and facility readiness scores (complete data set), and were included in the analyses.

Table 3.3 shows the linear regression models using endline facility performance score as a continuous outcome. In both the simple and multiple linear regression models, while the mean endline facility performance score increased for every 1 unit increase in the facility readiness score, this association was not statistically significant. The multiple regression models controlled for baseline facility performance score, mean delivery volume, and the level or type of health facilities.

Table 3.4 shows the results from multinomial logistic regression analyses which used tertiles of the endline facility performance score as categories. The mean endline facility performance score for the lowest tertile (n=45) was 4.96; that for the middle tertile (n=45) was 6.17; and for the highest tertile (n=44) was 7.18. The lowest tertile was used as the reference category. One unit increase in the facility readiness score was found to be associated with 0.51 unit increase (p=0.045) in the relative log odds of being in the middle vs. lowest tertile of the endline facility performance score, after controlling for baseline facility performance score, mean delivery volume, and the facility level. The beta coefficient (log odds) was exponentiated to obtain the odds ratio, which allows an easier and linear interpretation. With increasing facility readiness score, the odds of a facility being in the middle tertile of the endline facility performance score relative to the lowest tertile was 1.68 (95% CI = 1.02, 2.76),after controlling for baseline facility performance score, mean delivery volume, and the facility level. However, such a significant association was not found between the facility readiness score and being in the highest vs. lowest

tertile of endline facility performance score.

Table 3.3: Linear regression analysis with endline facility performance score as the dependent outcome

	Coefficient	standard error	95% CI of coefficient	p-value
Simple Linear Regression Model (n=132)				
Facility readiness score	0.15	0.09	-0.04, 0.33	0.111
Multiple Linear Regression Model 1 (n=132)				
Facility readiness score	0.19	0.1	-0.008, 0.40	0.059
Baseline facility performance score	0.12	0.07	-0.03, 0.26	0.11
Mean delivery volume	0.0005	0.0006	-0.0007, 0.002	0.394
Facility Level	-0.6	0.42	-1.44, 0.24	0.157
Multiple Linear Regression Model 2 (n=132)				
Facility readiness score	0.15	0.1	-0.05, 0.35	0.136
Baseline facility performance score	0.14	0.07	-0.008, 0.28	0.065
Mean delivery volume	0.00009	0.0006	-0.001, 0.001	0.884
Facility Type	-0.05	0.5	-1.05, 0.94	0.915

Note: Mean delivery volume reflects the average monthly facility-level delivery volume for 2019, based on CFA 2019 data.
Legends: MNC: maternal & newborn care; Facility Level: Level 2 or 3; CI: confidence interval; Facility Type: BEmONC/ CEmONC

Table 3.4: Multinomial logistic regression analysis with endline facility performance score tertiles as dependent outcome

	Coefficient	standard error	95% CI of coefficient	p-value
Simple Model (n=132)				
Endline performance score - lowest tertile	Reference			
Endline performance score - middle tertile				
Facility readiness score	0.17	0.22	-0.25, 0.60	0.423
Endline performance score - highest tertile				
Facility readiness score	0.23	0.22	-0.20, 0.66	0.298
Multiple Multinomial Model 1 (n=132), model significant (p=0.0433)				
Endline performance score - lowest tertile	Reference			
Endline performance score - middle tertile				
Facility readiness score	**0.51**	**0.26**	**0.01, 1.01**	**0.045**
Baseline facility performance score	-0.09	0.17	-0.42, 0.25	0.612
Mean delivery volume	0.001	0.002	-0.002, 0.005	0.439
Facility Level	-3.7	1.45	-6.53, -0.86	**0.011**
Endline performance score - highest tertile				
Facility readiness score	0.39	0.25	-0.11, 0.88	0.128
Baseline facility performance score	0.24	0.19	-0.14, 0.62	0.213
Mean delivery volume	0.001	0.001	-0.001, 0.004	0.335
Facility Level	-1.52	1.02	-3.51, 0.48	0.137

Continued

	Coefficient	standard error	95% CI of coefficient	p-value
Multiple Multinomial Model 2 (n=132)				
Endline performance score - lowest tertile	Reference			
Endline performance score - middle tertile				
Facility readiness score	0.33	0.24	-0.14, 0.80	0.171
Baseline facility performance score	-0.02	0.16	-0.34, 0.30	0.89
Mean delivery volume	-0.0003	0.002	-0.004, 0.003	0.866
Facility Type	-1.81	1.44	-4.62, 1.004	0.208
Endline performance score - highest tertile				
Facility readiness score	0.22	0.24	-0.25, 0.70	0.361
Baseline facility performance score	0.31	0.19	-0.07, 0.68	0.108
Mean delivery volume	0.00001	0.001	-0.003, 0.003	0.993
Facility Type	0.2	1.1	-1.96, 2.36	0.855

Note: Mean delivery volume reflects the average monthly facility-level delivery volume for 2019, based on CFA 2019 data.
Legends: MNC: maternal & newborn care; Facility Level: Level 2 or 3; CI: confidence interval; Facility Type: BEmONC/ CEmONC

3.4 Discussion

The BTSP focused on improving RMNCH program outcomes in Bihar through identifying and addressing bottlenecks across the health system and functionalizing all public health facilities which conducted deliveries – a good example of the diagonal approach to health system strengthening. It embarked on a twin strategy to achieve this goal –addressing gaps in infrastructure, supply chain, and human resources to improve the facility readiness, as well as mentoring the ANM and GNM nurses to improve the quality of service delivery, and therefore, the facility-level performance. This dual approach was deemed necessary to achieve sustainable improvement in the coverage and quality of RMNCH services in the long run. While earlier publications had examined the successes and shortcomings of these two interventions separately, the current paper aimed to examine if these two initiatives were supporting and associated with each other, given the limitations of available data. The analysis focused on 2 main aspects – the relative improvement in facility performance before and after the AMANAT *Jyoti* intervention, and the complex relationship between facility readiness and facility performance. Improvements were noted for 36 (80%) of the 45 parameters assessed through direct observation of deliveries between the baseline and endline, and the mean facility performance score increased significantly among both levels (Level 2 and 3) and both types (BEmONC and CEmONC) of facilities. However, the analysis failed to identify a linear relationship between facility readiness and facility performance scores, while a significant positive association was observed between the facility readiness score and the middle tertile of endline facility performance score (vs. lowest tertile as reference) in multiple multinomial logistic regression modeling. While there is no doubt that the relationship between facility readiness and facility performance is a nuanced one, the following sections attempt to present a sequential interpretation of these complex

findings, and their implications for improving Bihar's public health system.

3.4.1 The relative improvement in quality of care through AMANAT *Jyoti*

The current paper found that the AMANAT *Jyoti* nurse-mentoring intervention had a positive

impact on improving the majority of observed practices while conducting deliveries and caring

for the newborn. However, as discussed earlier, the AMANAT *Jyoti* is essentially a modified

continuation of the AMANAT interventions initiated between 2015 and 2017, and the mobile

nurse mentoring program before that (2012-2014). Thus, the baseline assessment results

essentially represent performance of the public health nursing cadre after several rounds of

periodic onsite mentoring. In that light, at least 80% compliance was observed for only 11 (24%)

of the assessed parameters at baseline, and 16 (36%) at endline. Hence, while interpreting the

relative improvement in assessment parameters (presented in Table 3.1), one needs to be

cognizant of the overall low level of provider compliance with these basic and critical steps for

managing normal deliveries and providing care to the newborn, including addressing immediate

emergencies like postpartum hemorrhage and birth asphyxia.

3.4.1.1 Maternal care provision

Among the parameters assessed to understand the quality of care provided to pregnant women in

the labor rooms, 90% (or more) compliance was noted at the endline for conducting pre-delivery

vaginal examination, post-delivery genital tract exploration, and avoiding mistakes like injecting

oxytocin before the third stage of labor, giving fundal pressure anytime during the labor, or

doing post-delivery vaginal packing. Remarkable improvements were noted in the practices of

giving counter cord traction (in 82% instances at endline, a 26 percentage-points improvement)

and uterine massages (in 88% instances at endline, a 37 percentage-points improvement).

Immediate initiation of intravenous fluids and injecting a loading dose of oxytocin was correctly done in 80% of the patients diagnosed with postpartum hemorrhage at the endline. On the other hand, concerns remained with less-than-50% compliance – even at the endline – with basic steps like measuring pre-delivery or post-delivery maternal blood pressure, pulse and temperature, as well as conducting pre-delivery abdominal examination or monitoring fetal heart rate. A notable decline (by 14 percentage-points) in performance was observed in administering oxytocin for active management of the third stage of labor – this step was performed during 37% of the endline observations. Despite improvement from baseline, only 27% of all episiotomies were clinically indicated, perineal support was not given during 70% of deliveries, and 74% of the episiotomy incisions and/or vaginal tears were not repaired. Only one-fifth of the delivery attendants washed their hands with soap and water during the endline assessments, while sterile instrument sets were used in only 60% of the deliveries – signaling a persistent threat to infection prevention inside the labor rooms.

Analysis of the quality of service delivery in 905 health facilities in Tanzania[100] with regards to performing the 7 WHO BEmONC signal functions revealed a comparable picture – while appreciable compliance was noted for some parameters, the opposite was observed for others. For example, while 83% of facilities reported that they parenterally administered oxytocin, only 34% did so for antibiotics and 13% for anticonvulsants. Nearly 70% of facilities conducted assisted vaginal delivery, but less than 36% reported manually removing placenta and/or the retained products of conception. Further, little over half the facilities reported performing neonatal resuscitation. In perspective, less than 30% of these facilities scored 50% on service readiness that was assessed based on staff availability and training, availability of equipment and essential supplies – indicating a lack of structural and technical support in meeting the minimum quality criteria. Researchers in Ghana[114] measured the quality of care in labor and in the immediate postpartum period based on defined signal functions, and found that 63% of the 64 assessed delivery points could not perform at least 4 out of 8 emergency obstetric care signal functions, 58% could not perform at least 3 out of 6 emergency newborn care signal functions, while about 60% could not perform 6 of the 12 routine labor care signal functions. In many cases, absence of the minimum number of skilled providers was associated with poor facility-level performance. Overall, only 18% facilities could be identified with satisfactory quality scores in all the studied dimensions. Bedoya et. al[115] observed infection prevention and control practices among health workers at over 900 primary care facilities in Kenya, and found that the mean compliance with standard, evidence-based guidelines was about 32%. The compliance was poorest for following hand hygiene measures (23%) while appreciable for intravenous procedures (87%). Further, hand hygiene practices remained poor even in the facilities with running water and handwashing supplies. This is a notable finding for the BTSP, since it signals that despite presence of infrastructure, adopting safe, hygienic behavior remains a challenge among frontline healthcare workers.

3.4.1.2 Newborn care provision

In the current analysis, among the parameters assessed to evaluate provider performance in essential newborn care, near-universal compliance was observed at the endline with regards to avoiding application of any ointment (or otherwise) on the cord stump, recording birth weight, and registering the birth in facility records. A number of practices like immediately drying the newborn and covering with a clean cloth, checking the cord for pulsations before clamping, delaying the clamping, using sterile material to tie and sterile scissors to cut the cord, as well as ensuring skin-to-skin contact within 5 minutes of delivery and initiating breastfeeding within an hour – mostly improved (by 4-40 percentage-points) from the baseline. However, the overall level of compliance with any of these parameters remained between 65-75% of the observed instances at endline. Wiping the newborns' eyes with sterile wet gauze remained poorly complied with – done in only 20% of the observations at endline. Marked deterioration was noted in the practices while managing birth asphyxia. Suction/ stimulation was provided in only about 72% of the required cases (15 percentage-points decrease) at endline. Poor compliance with this key step seemingly negated the 13 percentage-points improvement achieved in the proportion of cases (87%) where post-suction bag-and-mask ventilation was needed and done. As a consequence, the overall performance in stabilizing such asphyxiated newborns within the facility declined – more than 50% of these babies could not be managed within the facility and had to be referred (17 percentage-points deterioration from baseline).

Comparable results had been reported from an assessment of the quality of newborn care services in Ethiopia, Kenya, Madagascar, Mozambique, Rwanda and Tanzania[116] through direct observation of antenatal care and labor practices. Across the countries, 94% of the deliveries observed involved cutting the cord with clean blades, and in nearly 80% of cases the babies were immediately dried after birth. However, less than 45% of all mothers were supported by the providers to initiate breast feeding within 1 hour post-delivery, or to initiate kangaroo mother care. Handwashing prior to conducting the deliveries was observed in only 37% of cases. Among the 209 babies born with asphyxia, 49% did not receive any intervention in the form of stimulation or head positioning to ensure open airways. Simulated assessment (with *NeoNatalie* models) of provider competency to conduct neonatal resuscitation in Madagascar, Rwanda and Tanzania demonstrated that only between one-fourth to one-third of all providers in each country could successfully perform all the necessary steps.

3.4.1.3 Key messages for future

Evidence from the current analysis, in-sync with findings from the literature, clearly signals the challenges in ensuring provider compliance with the most basic and critical steps in preventing maternal and neonatal morbidity and mortality. Similar results had been observed during assessments of the previous versions of AMANAT, as mentioned earlier. While the pre- and post-intervention assessments had consistently found significant improvement in knowledge and practices among the mentored nurses,[22, 68-70, 111] the overall performance (like the proportion of essential tasks successfully completed) had remained low and often deteriorated[70, 112] over the next 1 year. Hence, in the current paper, though the mentored nurses in Bihar demonstrated improvement in their performance across the majority of the 45 assessed parameters, the results can hardly be a source of satisfaction.

Consequently, the findings not only necessitate continuing AMANAT *Jyoti* mentoring as a regular, system-driven process in the foreseeable future, but also call for possible institutionalized efforts that would optimize and sustain the desired quality of care in service delivery. There are several successful examples from the IFHI (2011-2013) phase that can be readily incorporated into the current program. First, a mobile app-based platform – similar to the one developed through the CARE-Dimagi partnership and piloted among frontline health workers[46] – can potentially become a valuable resource for the nurses. This app can be used to make job aids and tools readily accessible to the nurses, while also providing a scope to perform self-assessments through charting/ documentation, while providing MNC services. Previously, such mobile-based apps were shown to be associated with increased home visits by the frontline workers and likely influenced better breastfeeding practices.[48, 50-52] Second, facility-based platforms can be created to provide opportunity to the nurses to engage in weekly sharing of challenges and best practices, especially in presence of a supervisor who can provide necessary guidance. During the IFHI phase, such clinic-levels gatherings were utilized to implement a "team-based goals and incentives" program under which the entire team of frontline workers would be rewarded (non-monetary incentives) if the clinic achieved a set of pre-determined targets.[46, 48, 49] The frontline workers participating in this program reported improved team-coordination, job satisfaction from public appreciation of their work, and perception of empowerment – and these factors were found to be more motivating than the incentives.[55, 56] This provides sufficient justification to implement the "team-based goals and incentives" program for the mentored nurses at the facility-level. Finally, periodic, active monitoring of the quality of service provision needs to be conducted by district-level and/or block-level quality assurance teams – to ensure that adhering to standard practices becomes a routine during day-to-day work. BTSP's health governance structure already includes district quality assurance committees in all 38 districts[63] – and these could be specifically charged with overseeing the periodic quality inspections to improve and sustain facility performance.

3.4.2 The complex relationship between facility readiness and performance

In the current analysis, the mean facility performance score increased significantly between baseline and endline assessments for both levels (Level 2 and 3) and both types (BEmONC and CEmONC) of facilities. However, what stands out from the results in Table 3.2 is the fact that the mean facility performance score remained higher for Level 2 and BEmONC facilities both at baseline and endline compared to Level 3 and CEmONC facilities. Since all facilities were assessed on 45 common parameters that involved managing normal delivery and providing essential newborn care (with immediate complications), it can certainly be said that the nurses at Level 2/ BEmONC facilities demonstrated much better performance over their counterparts at higher-level institutions. However, the Level 3 and CEmONC facilities did show greater improvement (endline–baseline mean difference), but it is difficult to draw conclusions due to the small sample size (Level 3: n=13; CEmONC: n=9). In contrast, the mean facility readiness score was, as expected, higher for Level 3 and CEmONC facilities. These facilities – the sub-divisional and district hospitals – are typically better equipped with the basic resources assessed in Panel 3.2 and manage twice the average delivery volume compared to lower-level facilities. Though the summary analysis in Table 3.2 provided an early indication of the discordance between the two scores, the regression analyses in Tables 3.3 and 3.4 provided deeper insights. The simple and multiple linear regressions failed to identify any statistically significant association between the endline facility performance and facility readiness scores. However, the multiple multinomial logistic regression analysis found that with increasing facility readiness score, the odds of a facility being in the middle tertile of the endline facility performance score relative to the lowest tertile was 1.68 (95% CI = 1.02, 2.76), after controlling for baseline facility performance score, mean delivery volume, and the facility level (but not the facility type). In simpler words, the model showed that there was a significant positive association between the endline facility performance and facility readiness scores, but this association was limited to the middle tertile of the endline facility performance score, when compared with the lowest tertile. No association was found for the highest vs. lowest tertiles of the endline facility performance score.

While the presence of adequate health workforce, basic infrastructure and essential supplies are deemed essential for facilities to deliver quality health care services, the mere presence of these inputs do not guarantee the desired outcome. Indeed, there has been evidence to the contrary, demonstrating that the quality of care received by patients can remain compromised even in the presence of adequate inputs. A survey of 4354 health facilities in Haiti, Kenya, Malawi, Namibia, Rwanda, Senegal, Tanzania, and Uganda[117] indicated a weak association (median correlation = 0.20) between facility-level infrastructure and evidence-based care provision, and the findings varied widely even among facilities with similar levels of infrastructure. The study could not identify a "minimum level" of infrastructure that would predict quality-assured service provision. Kaur et. al[118] conducted a cross-sectional structural assessment of 190 primary health centers and 36 district hospitals of Bihar in 2016, and linked the findings with household-level maternal and child health survey data collected by CARE India during the same period. They constructed composite indices for facility-level structural capacity (based on infrastructure, equipment and medicines) and human resources availability, and tested their association with a patient-reported quality of care index based on 11 essential pre- and post-partum services. For the primary health centers, the study failed to find any association. However, at the level of district hospitals, a positive trend (not quantified) was observed between the human resources availability and quality of care indices.

The current analysis compared two scores that were developed on a number of parameters which complemented each other – 44 facility readiness parameters covering the availability of human resources, labor room infrastructure and essential supplies (equipment, medicines, commodities), which were needed to perform the 45 parameters on which the mentored nurses were assessed through direct observation of deliveries and newborn care practices. While theoretically these two scores may be expected to be positively associated, in practice, the relationship is far more nuanced. Though there remains no critical threshold level for facility readiness, it may be rationally argued that the presence of all 44 indicators used to construct the current facility readiness score remain the minimum essential requirement in any MNC service delivery setting.

In the same breath, any effort to address the quality of MNC services needs to guarantee compliance with most, if not all of the 45 performance parameters observed.

Qualitative studies involving AMANAT mentors (2015-2017) had previously highlighted the existing infrastructural and supply chain obstacles faced by the mentee nurses while providing urgent obstetric and neonatal care. Physical distance between the labor room and the newborn care corner, along with shortages in availability of functional autoclaves, mucous extractors, oxygen and ventilation bags made it very challenging for the overburdened nurses to manage obstetric emergencies or neonatal resuscitations. In many cases, even basic equipment like gloves and intravenous catheters, and essential medicines like antibiotics, uterotonics and antihypertensives were in short supply; whereas absence of properly-equipped ambulances limited the ability to arrange effective referrals.[69, 119, 120] Based on the analysis of CFA 2019 data presented in the second paper of this book, some of these gaps – like the availability of ambulances and relocation of newborn care corners inside the labor rooms – had remarkably improved by 2019. However, the same assessment also identified that basic equipment like stethoscopes and blood pressure instruments were still not present in nearly 40% of labor rooms, at least one among functional autoclave/ electric sterilizer/ boiler was not present in nearly 50% of labor rooms, and functional oxygen cylinders were not present in over 60% labor rooms. CFA 2019 further demonstrated persistent weaknesses in the supply chain system that led to stock-outs of normal saline and Ringer's lactate solutions, basic consumables like cotton and gauze rolls, personal protective gear (caps, face masks, gloves), intravenous cannulas and syringes, urinary catheters and urine collection bags. 50% of all facilities could not provide a clean towel for the newborn, and 75% could not provide gowns for the pregnant women in labor. It thus becomes clear that public health facilities in Bihar are quite some distance away from meeting

the minimum essential requirements to ensure quality MNC service delivery.

Health system assessments in Ghana[93, 121] and Tanzania[122] had revealed that the lack of training

and/or experience among physician and non-physician cadres to correctly use appropriate

equipment and essential supplies, and perform one or more of the 7 WHO BEmONC signal

functions often contributed to poor quality clinical management of pregnant women. One-off

training courses involving midwives and nurses had insignificant impact. Additionally, the lack

of adequate infrastructure and supplies often made the situation worse. A recent systematic

review of midwifery services in India noted that while lack of professional competency along

with poorly equipped public health facilities negatively impacted the quality of care provided by

these health workers, periodic hands-on training programs together with a supportive system for

supervision enabled better job performance.[79] Helfinstein et. al[123] studied the relative importance

of skilled providers (nursing staff) versus the facilities in ensuring quality of care provided to

pregnant women in labor. They utilized data from 244 community and primary health centers in

Uttar Pradesh state of India (on the number of vital signs assessed during labor), along with

nationally representative data from Kenya and Malawi (to estimate respectful and competent care

delivery). Through a variance decomposition analysis, the researchers found that facilities, rather

than the nurses, played a dominant role in determining the quality of care received by a patient.

In fact, facilities accounted for 3-10 times more variance in quality of care. In other words, while

the quality of care provided by all nurses within a particular facility were more likely to be at

par, that between individual facilities could vary substantially. The paper concluded that it was

more important to focus on holistic improvement of a health facility through strengthening

infrastructure and supplies as well as training the providers present, rather than spending resources on solely addressing provider skills and behavior, especially for providing care that did not warrant sophisticated instrumentation or specialized training (like labor room services). The results from the current paper resonate with these findings from India and around the developing world. They offer some indication that the facility-level health system strengthening work in Bihar is likely on the right trajectory, but this comes with a strong caveat – that the BTSP must strive more to accomplish a level where these two facility-level interventions would strongly complement each other and indeed make a difference in population health outcomes. It is in this perspective that the results from the current analysis may be best interpreted for program and policy purposes.

3.4.3 Limitations

The current study relied on analysis of existing programmatic data that was generated through facility-level assessments of structural readiness (CFA 2019) and MNC service delivery performance (2018-19 AMANAT *Jyoti* assessment) conducted by CARE India's CML Unit. Though the AMANAT *Jyoti* program is being implemented in over 350 facilities, the paper could only utilize the pre- and post-intervention data available from 134 health facilities due to operational reasons. Consequently, there was a limitation of sample size, and it particularly affected analyzing progress in Level 3 (n=13) and CEmONC (n=9) health facilities. It is also quite likely that this limitation affected results of the regression analyses, and hence the paper adopted caution in interpreting the same.

Second, the two scores compared in this paper were developed from two different surveys. While the CFA 2019 (conducted August-September 2019) immediately preceded the endline AMANAT *Jyoti* assessment (conducted in October-December 2019), it would have been preferable to have the facility readiness and facility performance data generated through a single assessment (or through 2 concurrent assessments). The availability status for functional equipment and essential supplies can change over a short period of time, and these changes can bias the true relationship between facility readiness and facility performance scores in either direction. Further, concurrent assessment can potentially reduce any temporal changes which may introduce bias – for example, the limitations of transport during the rainy season that can hamper the availability of essential supplies. However, these are common limitations of working with field-level data that is generated for the purposes of routinely monitoring and evaluating progress and is not collected for research purposes.

Third, while the regression analyses controlled for some potential measured confounders like the baseline facility performance score, there are more complexities to consider. It is quite likely that a number of nurses at baseline may not have gone through all or any of the previous rounds of AMANAT interventions. Similarly, there's no way to verify if all nurses observed at endline had actually undergone the baseline AMANAT *Jyoti* training. These issues call for a mixed-methods process evaluation to be in-built in subsequent iterations of AMANAT *Jyoti*, to help understand the formative shortcomings during implementation, assess the quality of training offered, and gain better perspectives regarding the outcomes. Unless this heterogeneity is captured, it would be difficult to understand if the change in facility performance score is truly attributable to the AMANAT *Jyoti* intervention, especially in absence of a control group.

Finally, construction of the facility performance score, just like the facility readiness score (as explained in the second paper of this book), did not follow the standard statistical procedures that would otherwise be warranted to create a complex, nuanced index reflecting the overall facility-level performance. While accepting this limitation, it is also important to point out that the facility performance score was developed as an operational score to capture the changes in facility performance (Panel 3.2) corresponding to the changes in facility readiness (Panel 3.1). The selection of 45 parameters to construct this score was done on the basis of repeated consultations between stakeholders who represented the government and its development partners. Hence, this score provides a summary understanding of the progress in facility performance, and its scope remains limited to understanding the program in Bihar. In sync with the facility readiness score, the facility performance score shall be expanded in future to measure progress in service areas beyond MNC.

3.5 Conclusion

The BTSP had strategized to concurrently work on expanding service coverage for RMNCH through structurally strengthening the public health facilities across Bihar, while also focusing on improving the quality of care. The current paper found that this dual approach was well-grounded in evidence, though the results certainly indicated towards an ongoing, unfinished project. While the performance of mentored nurses improved through the AMANAT *Jyoti* intervention, the overall level of compliance with basic and critical steps to ensure maternal and neonatal wellbeing remained unacceptably low. The results also did not point towards reassuring evidence that facility readiness was associated with facility performance. However, this lack of evidence was most likely due to the persistent challenges faced by Bihar's public health facilities in meeting the minimum requirements for infrastructure and supplies, and the known difficulties in modifying behaviors and practices of frontline health care workers who are expected to perform within the existing limitations of these facilities and cater to high patient volumes. The second paper of this book had previously recommended that BTSP should prioritize addressing the remaining infrastructural gaps like ensuring adequate handwashing stations (with running water and soap) and labor tables through targeted public funding and setting time-bound block- and district-level goals. Further, the BTSP also needed to disentangle supply-chain issues at the facility level, preferably through implementing electronic/ web-based systems for managing inventory and training the designated personnel to use such systems correctly and efficiently.

Regarding the AMANAT *Jyoti* intervention, while the sub-par performance of the nurses at Level 3/ CEmONC facilities was a concerning finding, it is difficult to recommend specific program modifications due to the small sample size at this level. However, the BTSP should look to re-conduct this analysis once the data from all/ majority of the 350+ facilities are available, and that would help gain deeper understanding of the comparative effectiveness of AMANAT *Jyoti* in BEmONC vs. CEmONC or Level 2 vs. Level 3 facilities.

A resonating message that emerges from the current analysis and evidence-based discussion is the need to realize that the challenges faced by BTSP are not unique in the context of resource-poor national/ sub-national health systems. There is an unquestionable need to continue addressing the structural shortcomings in Bihar's public health facilities, while also ensuring that the AMANAT *Jyoti* becomes a regular, system-driven training program that covers all current and newly-inducted nurses. Additional factors that drive and sustain high levels of performance and improve workforce motivation such as mobile app-based job aids and tools, team-based goals and incentives programs, as well as active, periodic monitoring of the quality of service provision by district- and/or block-level quality assurance teams should also be considered. Developing a cluster of facilities as models to test the effectiveness and inter-relationship of this dual strategy might be a pragmatic approach to quantitatively demonstrate that improvements in facility readiness and facility performance can positively and significantly support each other. The results from the current paper provide hopeful indications towards that end. Further, such evidence might be useful in securing long-term funding support for the BTSP from Gates Foundation, as well as motivate the government policymakers to actively engage in accelerating progress in expanding RMNCH service coverage and improving the quality of service delivery.

Conclusion

The Bihar Technical Support Program (BTSP) is an important diagonal health system strengthening initiative – one that starts with a focus on specific programmatic (RMNCH) outcomes, but strives to achieve these through identifying and addressing bottlenecks across the health system. Such an approach maximizes the utilization of existing health system resources through synchronizing vertical health programs and horizontal systemic interventions. Further, it can potentially make gains in population health outcomes sustainable, particularly when supported by purposeful health governance and efficient public financing, even in the absence of external support.[75]

Since its inception in November 2013, BTSP has helped develop a novel structure of health governance whereby state-, district- and block-level technical support teams were created and fully embedded within the state health system. This was necessary to co-develop health system interventions with the state government, and transfer ownership of the implementation and monitoring activities. Equally significant was the capacity building in collecting and using facility-level data to inform programs and policies. The book has shown that BTSP has made appreciable progress in structurally preparing Bihar's Level 2 and Level 3 public health facilities (facility readiness) to deliver basic maternal and newborn care (MNC) services – with improvements in related infrastructure, essential supplies, and supportive services like referral transport and laboratory facilities, as well as through recruitment of large number of ANM and GNM nurses. In spite of this success, some serious shortcomings remained across these areas, which could potentially impede continued progress.

While the concurrent nurse-mentoring initiative (AMANAT *Jyoti*) contributed to relative improvement in facility performance (quality of service delivery), as evidenced by the baseline-endline assessment differential, challenges persist that could threaten these positive trends. The overall level of provider compliance with basic and critical steps to ensure maternal and neonatal wellbeing still remained unacceptably low. It is worth remembering that the parameters used to construct the facility readiness and performance scores truly represent a set of basic minimum requirements in structural capability and quality of care. Hence, the limited evidence of a significant positive association between endline facility performance and facility readiness scores is rather a testimony to the modest levels of facility readiness and facility performance achieved by Bihar's public health facilities to date. Consequently, it is imperative for BTSP to continue addressing the persistent challenges in facility readiness and facility performance, so that these two facility-level interventions will complement each other and influence outcomes in the near future.

1. Implications for BTSP

Successive comprehensive facility assessments (CFAs, 2015-2019) have identified 3 major issues which currently impede facility readiness to provide MNC services, and warrant immediate attention. First, it is important to ensure that the basic minimum infrastructure to provide MNC services is developed and maintained at all public health facilities. Fundamental amenities like functional handwashing stations (with running water and soap), adequate labor tables, and appropriate sanitation systems are indispensable for ensuring proper service provision. The BTSP may want to prioritize such deficiencies, streamline necessary funding through the Bihar Medical Services & Infrastructure Corporation Limited, and set time-bound targets for the block- and district-level health administrations.

Second, while the supply chain system does depend on macro-issues like state-level funding and centralized procurement and distribution, the current analysis revealed a major deficiency in scaling-up of the facility-level electronic/ web-based inventory-management system (*e-Aushadhi*). As of 2019, only 41% of the surveyed facilities had this software, and most of the drug storage room supervisors were not trained to use this system correctly and efficiently. Erroneous stock-in (or stock-out) status of the supplies in the software potentially compromised the procurement and distribution system at the facility and district levels. The BTSP may want to focus on ensuring rapid scale-up of this inventory management system in all facilities, along with hands-on training programs aimed at capacity building, before the next CFA. Periodic monitoring of facility-level utilization of *e-Aushadhi* could be done by block and district level teams to incentivize compliance during the early years.

Third, while shortage of specialist physicians in public health facilities is a common problem in India's public health system, BTSP may want to explore the "task shifting" approach[109] to rationally redistribute specific roles to the available workforce of nurses and primary care physicians. This shall require setting up of hub-and-spoke models to implement tailor-made training programs, and the process may be best implemented at the district-level – with district hospitals serving as hubs (centralized resources) and peripheral health facilities participating as spokes. There is ample evidence that task shifting not only makes efficient use of the available human resources, but also ensures and indeed improves the quality of care provision.[110] CFA 2019 has demonstrated that a large number of ANM nurses are already available at all facilities, and this creates a good basis to implement the task shifting approach.

The findings from the assessment of BTSP's nurse mentoring program – AMANAT *Jyoti*, in sync with the published literature on previous versions of AMANAT, clearly demonstrated the challenges in ensuring provider compliance with the most basic and critical steps in preventing maternal and neonatal morbidity and mortality. While the pre- and post-intervention assessments had consistently found significant performance improvements among the mentored nurses, the overall performance (like the proportion of essential tasks successfully completed) had remained low, and often deteriorated over the subsequent year. There is enough evidence from low and middle income countries demonstrating that despite the presence of infrastructure, adopting safe, hygienic behavior remains a challenge among frontline healthcare workers – and the system must ensure repetitive cycles of training over sufficient time to inculcate such good practices as routine. Thus, there is a clear need to continue AMANAT *Jyoti* as a regular, system-driven training program in the foreseeable future to gradually develop competency among both current (in-service training) and newly-inducted (pre-service training) nurses. Additional factors that drive and sustain high levels of performance and improve workforce motivation such as mobile app-based job aids and tools, team-based goals and incentives programs, as well as active, periodic monitoring of the quality of service provision by district- and/or block-level quality assurance teams should also be considered. Linking participation in the mentoring programs and subsequent performance to career progression goals may offer a long-term solution to incentivize the nursing cadre. Further, a mixed-methods process evaluation should be incorporated into subsequent iterations of AMANAT *Jyoti*, to help understand the formative shortcomings during implementation, assess the quality of training offered, and gain better perspectives regarding the outcomes. In-depth interviews and/or focus group discussions with the AMANAT mentors as well as the mentee nurses would certainly contribute to deeper understanding of the challenges in ensuring change in provider behaviors and practices. The BTSP may also consider formulating a holistic MNC training program that incorporates both management procedures (written policy, staff training, regular monitoring) and clinical practices (correct procedures and client education), much in-line with the WHO/ UNICEF Baby Friendly Hospital Initiative.[124]

2. Implications for health systems research

A key finding from this book was the absence of reassuring evidence that facility readiness was positively and significantly associated with facility performance. While the lack of adequate progress among Bihar's public health facilities in these two dimensions (readiness and performance) may be the potential reason behind this finding, it may also be helpful to design a study to take a deeper dive. Developing a cluster of facilities (in a particular district) as models to test the effectiveness and inter-relationship of this dual strategy might be a pragmatic approach to quantitatively demonstrate that improvements in facility readiness and facility performance can positively and significantly support each other. Such evidence might be useful in demonstrating the true utility of this health system strengthening approach to both the funder (Gates Foundation) and the government policymakers, and secure long-term commitments.

In the same context, it may be necessary to address the methodological shortcomings arising from assessing facility readiness and facility performance through two separate surveys and over different time-periods. The availability status for functional equipment and essential supplies can change over a short period of time, and these changes can bias the true relationship between facility readiness and facility performance scores in either direction. Further, considerable attention is also required to develop more sensitive assessment tools to evaluate facility readiness and facility performance, and explore if different statistical weightage may be accorded to some structural parameters and performance steps.

3. Implications for public policymakers

The facility-level assessments from Bihar as well as from similar other settings convey a common message – that a health system strengthening approach to achieve program outcomes often requires more time to show results, as the path traverses through the challenging terrains of improving infrastructure, addressing supply chain complexities, and recruiting skilled human resource for health. Consequently, it remains important to appreciate the complexity of this process. This consideration assumes further importance based on the fact that the evolution of BTSP represented a critical transformation of the collaborative approach between the Bihar government and its development partners.

Under BTSP, the state health system gradually assumed a more dominant role in program implementation, while the development partners were relegated to providing technical and managerial assistance. There are fundamental differences in service delivery approaches between a development partner and a government, likely attributable to the differences in organizational culture.[104] Hence, in all fairness, the Bihar government should be accorded more time to fully integrate all interventions within its own system, and premature conclusions on the lack of rapid improvements may be unjust. It had been observed that prolonged periods of intensive program implementation directly by external partners can actually do more harm than good to a local public health system – as the latter has no incentive to own the development process and improve from within.[105] The BTSP and the Bihar government may do well to appreciate and address the challenges during this transitional phase, specifically in sharing ownership of the gaps in implementation, and shouldering the responsibility for outcomes. This will be critical to future success of the overall health system strengthening program. Additionally, the Bihar government should consider taking steps to generate demand for health services through outreach activities, as community engagement can serve as a strong stimulus to accelerate facility readiness and performance.

It is encouraging to note that the funding support for BTSP is being continued, and the state health policymakers may seek to utilize this period to proactively engage in assuming increasing responsibility – and this would define the long-term sustainability of the current efforts. This book identified myriad challenges on the road ahead, yet found evidence to hope that purposeful improvements would go a long way to create a more efficient, sustainable, and equitable public health system in Bihar.

4. A last word

The long shadow of the COVID-19 pandemic was cast on the entire lifespan of this book – starting from finalization of the protocol in July, 2020 to the defense in August, 2021. Fortunately, the candidate and the CARE India Bihar team had accounted for some of the subsequent unforeseen disruptions during the protocol planning stages, ably supported by a responsive supervisory committee.

Consequent to the travel restrictions between USA and India at different points of time, as well as the periodic lockdowns in India, the entire research work had to be conducted remotely. This not only complicated the entire process, but also imposed limitations on planning further steps which could have potentially enriched the research work – for example, conducting interviews and/ or focused group discussions with government officials and health workers in Bihar to gain additional insights into the evolution of the BTSP (Paper 1). Hence, the book research was limited to analyzing data that had already been generated (CFA 2015, 2016, 2017 and 2019; AMANAT *Jyoti* assessments, 2018-2019) and were readily available with the Concurrent Monitoring and Learning unit of CARE India, Patna office.

During this one year research period, members of the Bihar CARE India team were frequently called on to assist the state government in planning and implementing pandemic response measures. The team members travelled to remote areas and remained inaccessible for long periods of time. Thankfully, such obstacles did not preclude the rigorous data analysis and periodic communications between the candidate and the CARE India Bihar team. The committee was appraised of the periodic progress and the dynamically evolving ground situation, and remained sensitive of these challenges while providing technical feedback on the research papers. This tripartite understanding of pandemic-imposed limitations and mutual roles immensely contributed to the successful completion of the current book.

References

1.   Reddy KS. India's Aspirations for Universal Health Coverage. *The New England journal of medicine*. Jul 2 2015;373(1):1-5. doi:10.1056/NEJMp1414214

2.   Angell BJ, Prinja S, Gupt A, Jha V, Jan S. The Ayushman Bharat Pradhan Mantri Jan Arogya Yojana and the path to universal health coverage in India: Overcoming the challenges of stewardship and governance. *PLoS medicine*. Mar 2019;16(3):e1002759. doi:10.1371/journal.pmed.1002759

3.   Ministry of Health & Family Welfare, Govt of India. National Health Accounts Estimates for India Financial Year 2015-16. National Health Systems Resource Centre; 2018. https://mohfw.gov.in/sites/default/files/NHA_Estimates_Report_2015-16.pdf

4.   Ministry of Health & Family Welfare GoI. *National Health Policy 2017*. 2017. Accessed January 30, 2018. https://mohfw.gov.in/sites/default/files/9147562941489753121.pdf

5.   Sangar S, Dutt V, Thakur R. Economic burden, impoverishment and coping mechanisms associated with out-of-pocket health expenditure: analysis of rural-urban differentials in India. journal article. *Journal of Public Health*. October 01 2018;26(5):485-494. doi:10.1007/s10389-018-0904-x

6.   KPMG (India). Healthcare: Union Budget 2017-18 Post-Budget sectoral point of view. July 22, 2018. Accessed July 22, 2018. https://home.kpmg.com/content/dam/kpmg/in/pdf/2017/02/Healthcare.pdf

7.   Karan A, Selvaraj S, Mahal A. Moving to universal coverage? Trends in the burden of out-of-pocket payments for health care across social groups in India, 1999-2000 to 2011-12. *PLoS One*. 2014;9(8):e105162. doi:10.1371/journal.pone.0105162

8.   World Health Organization. Global Health Observatory data repository: Under-5 mortality Data by urban wealth quintile. WHO. February 20, 2020. Accessed February 20, 2020. http://apps.who.int/gho/data/view.main.vEQU5MORTWQv?lang=en

9.   Govt of India. Report of the National Commission on Macroeconomics and Health. MoHFW. Accessed November 20, 2017. www.who.int/macrohealth/action/Report%20of%20the%20National%20Commission.pdf.

10.   The National Bureau of Asian Research. Healthcare in India: A Call for Innovative Reform - An Interview with Victoria Fan February 7, 2018. Accessed February 7, 2018. http://nbr.org/research/activity.aspx?id=298

11.   Office of the Registrar General & Census Commissioner (India). CENSUS OF INDIA 2011 - PROVISIONAL POPULATON TOTALS. Ministry of Home Affairs, GoI. March 25, 2019. Accessed March 25, 2019. http://censusindia.gov.in/2011-prov-results/data_files/bihar/Provisional%20Population%20Totals%202011-Bihar.pdf

12.   Udyog Mitra, Department of Industries, Government of Bihar. Priority Sectors: Healthcare April 10, 2019. Accessed April 10, 2019. http://www.udyogmitrabihar.in/priority-sectors/healthcare/

13.   Mathew S, Moore M. IDS Working Paper 366 State Incapacity by Design: Understanding the Bihar Story Institute of Development Studies, University of Sussex 2011. April 20, 2020. Accessed April 20 , 2020. https://onlinelibrary.wiley.com/doi/pdf/10.1111/j.2040-0209.2011.00366.x

14.   International Institute for Population Sciences (IIPS). National Family Health Survey, India. IIPS. April 20, 2020. Accessed April 20, 2020. http://rchiips.org/nfhs/

15.	Office of the Registrar General & Census Commissioner, Ministry of Home Affairs, Government of India. Sample Registration System (SRS) Bulletins. GoI. April 20, 2020. Accessed April 20, 2020. http://censusindia.gov.in/vital_statistics/SRS_Bulletins/Bulletins.html

16.	Information & Public Relations Department, Government of Bihar. Bihar Report Card 2015: Development with Justice. 2015. https://www.bvm.bihar.gov.in/reportcard

17.	Health Department, Government of Bihar. Annual Report 2011-12. 2012. http://health.bih.nic.in/Docs/Annual-Report-2011-12.pdf

18.	Bill & Melinda Gates Foundation. Where We Work: India Office: Key Regions. BMGF. April 20, 2020. Accessed April 20, 2020. https://www.gatesfoundation.org/Where-We-Work/India-Office/Key-Regions

19.	CARE India. Bihar Technical Support Programme. CARE India. April 20, 2020. Accessed April 20, 2020. https://www.careindia.org/project/technical-assistance-to-the-government-of-bihar-improving-health-nutrition-coverage-and-outcomes/

20.	CARE India. Integrated Family Health Initiative (IFHI): Catalyzing Change in Bihar, India CARE India. March 18, 2020. https://www.care.org/sites/default/files/documents/Bihar_final_0.pdf

21.	Government of India. Rural Health Statistics 2014-15. GoI. February 20, 2020. Accessed February 20, 2020. https://wcd.nic.in/sites/default/files/RHS_1.pdf

22.	Creanga AA, Jiwani S, Das A, et al. Using a mobile nurse mentoring and training program to address a health workforce capacity crisis in Bihar, India: Impact on essential intrapartum and newborn care practices. *Journal of global health*. Dec 2020;10(2):021009. doi:10.7189/jogh.10.021009

23.   Government of India. National Health Mission. April 20, 2020. Accessed April 20, 2020. http://nhm.gov.in/

24.   Berman P, Bhawalkar M, Jha R. *Tracking financial resources for primary health care in BIHAR, India*. 2017. *A report of the Resource Tracking and Management Project* Accessed February 5, 2020. https://cdn1.sph.harvard.edu/wp-content/uploads/sites/2031/2017/01/Tracking-financial-resources-for-primary-health-care-in-BIHAR-India.pdf

25.   World Bank. *Bihar: Poverty, Growth & Inequality*. 2016. Accessed February 20, 2020. http://documents.worldbank.org/curated/en/781181467989480762/pdf/105842-BRI-P157572-PUBLIC-Bihar-Proverty.pdf

26.   Kumar V, Singh P. Access to healthcare among the Empowered Action Group (EAG) states of India: Current status and impeding factors. *Natl Med J India*. Sep-Oct 2016;29(5):267-273.

27.   CARE India. Towards a Healthier Bihar. CARE India. April 18, 2020. Accessed April 18, 2020. https://www.careindia.org/bihar/

28.   CARE India. Bihar Technical Support Program (BTSP). *Resources and Publications: Health*. CARE India; 2016. November 10, 2016. April 20, 2020. https://www.careindia.org/wp-content/uploads/2017/06/Bihar-presentation_-CARE-Atlanta-20161110.pdf

29.   Kruk ME, Gage AD, Arsenault C, et al. High-quality health systems in the Sustainable Development Goals era: time for a revolution. *The Lancet Global health*. Nov 2018;6(11):e1196-e1252. doi:10.1016/s2214-109x(18)30386-3

30.   CARE India. Annual Report. *Resources and Publications: Annual Reports*. 2014. https://www.careindia.org/wp-content/uploads/2017/05/CARE-India-Annual-Report-2014.pdf

31.   CARE India. Annual Report. *Resources and Publications: Annual Reports*. 2016. https://www.careindia.org/wp-content/uploads/2017/05/CARE-India-Annual-report-2016-5mb.pdf

32.   CARE India. Annual Report. *Resources and Publications: Annual Reports*. 2017. https://www.careindia.org/wp-content/uploads/2018/03/CARE-annual-report-March-21-FINAL.pdf

33.   CARE India. Annual Report. *Resources and Publications: Annual Reports*. 2018. https://careindia.org/wp-content/uploads/2019/03/CareAnnualReport.pdf

34.   CARE India. Impact Report: 2014-16. *Resources and Publications: Impact Reports*. 2019. https://www.careindia.org/wp-content/uploads/2019/03/Impact-Report.pdf

35.   CARE India. SDG Impact Report: 2019. *Resources and Publications: Impact Reports*. 2019. https://www.careindia.org/wp-content/uploads/2019/09/SDG-Impact-Report-2019.pdf

36.   CARE India. Resources and Publications. CARE India. April 18, 2020. Accessed April 18, 2020. https://www.careindia.org/resources/health/

37.   Finance Department, Govt. of Bihar. White Paper on State Finances and Development. 2006. http://finance.bih.nic.in/Reports/FWP-English.pdf

38.   World Health Organization, UNFPA, UNICEF, Mailman School of Public Health - Averting Maternal Death and Disability (AMDD). *Monitoring emergency obstetric care: a handbook*. WHO; 2009:152. Accessed December 23, 2020. https://www.who.int/reproductivehealth/publications/monitoring/9789241547734/en/

39.   National Health Systems Resource Centre (Technical Support Institute with National Health Mission). National Quality Assurance Standards (NQAS) Govt. of India. March 25, 2019.

Accessed March 25, 2019. http://qi.nhsrcindia.org/cms-detail/national-quality-assurance-standards/MTAx

40.   Maternal Health Division, Ministry of Health & Family Welfare. Maternal and Newborn Health Toolkit. Govt. of India; 2013. March 25, 2019. Accessed March 25, 2019. http://nhsrcindia.org/sites/default/files/Maternal%20%20Newborn%20Health%20Toolkit.pdf

41.   StataCorp. Stata Statistical Software: Release 15. College Station, TX: StataCorp LLC.; 2017.

42.   National Health Mission, Ministry of Health and Family Welfare. Indian Public Health Standards - Revised Guidelines 2012. Government of India. May 14, 2020. Accessed May 14, 2020. https://nhm.gov.in/index1.php?lang=1&level=2&sublinkid=971&lid=154

43.   Darmstadt GL, Pepper KT, Ward VC, et al. Improving primary health care delivery in Bihar, India: Learning from piloting and statewide scale-up of Ananya. *Journal of global health*. Dec 2020;10(2):021001. doi:10.7189/jogh.10.021001

44.   Darmstadt GL. Learning from Ananya: Lessons for primary health care performance improvement. *Journal of global health*. Dec 2020;10(2):020356. doi:10.7189/jogh.10.020356

45.   World Bank. *Bihar: Towards a Development Strategy*. 2006. Accessed March 25, 2020. http://documents.worldbank.org/curated/en/624671468035374716/pdf/328190IN0Bihar1reportl1June200501PUBLIC1.pdf

46.   CARE India. Integrated Family Health Initiative: Program Summary. *Resources and Publications: Health*. CARE India; 2013. May, 2013. April 20, 2020. https://www.careindia.org/wp-content/uploads/2017/04/BIHAR_IFHI_Multipage_Screen_May-2013-1.pdf

47.	CARE India. Building Skills, Saving Lives: The Incremental Learning Approach. *Resources and Publications: Health*. CARE India; 2018. 2018. April 20, 2020. https://www.careindia.org/wp-content/uploads/2019/07/Bihar_1_REV_SCREEN.pdf

48.	Sridharan S, Rangarajan A, Manoranjini M, Sethi S. *Using Supply- and Demand-Side Strategies to Improve Maternal and Child Health in Bihar, India: Process Evaluation Findings*. 2014. December 5, 2014. Accessed April 21, 2020. https://www.mathematica.org/our-publications-and-findings/publications/using-supply-and-demand-side-strategies-to-improve-maternal-and-child-health-in-bihar-india

49.	CARE India. Working Better Together: Team-Based Goals and Incentives. *Resources and Publications: Health*. CARE India; 2018. 2018. April 20, 2020. https://www.careindia.org/wp-content/uploads/2019/07/Bihar_2_REV_SCREEN.pdf

50.	Das A, Mahapatra S, Sai Mala G, Chaudhuri I, Mahapatra T. Association of Frontline Worker-Provided Services with Change in Block-Level Complementary Feeding Indicators: An Ecological Analysis from Bihar, India. *PLoS One*. 2016;11(11):e0166511. doi:10.1371/journal.pone.0166511

51.	Das A, Chatterjee R, Karthick M, Mahapatra T, Chaudhuri I. The Influence of Seasonality and Community-Based Health Worker Provided Counselling on Exclusive Breastfeeding - Findings from a Cross-Sectional Survey in India. *PLoS One*. 2016;11(8):e0161186. doi:10.1371/journal.pone.0161186

52.	Borkum E, Rotz D, Rangarajan A, et al. *Midline findings from the evaluation of the Ananya program in Bihar*. 2014. December 12, 2014. Accessed April 21, 2020. https://www.mathematica.org/our-publications-and-findings/publications/midline-findings-from-the-evaluation-of-the-ananya-program-in-bihar

53.   Balakrishnan R, Gopichandran V, Chaturvedi S, Chatterjee R, Mahapatra T, Chaudhuri I. Continuum of Care Services for Maternal and Child Health using mobile technology - a health system strengthening strategy in low and middle income countries. *BMC Med Inform Decis Mak.* Jul 7 2016;16:84. doi:10.1186/s12911-016-0326-z

54.   Carmichael SL, Mehta K, Srikantiah S, et al. Use of mobile technology by frontline health workers to promote reproductive, maternal, newborn and child health and nutrition: a cluster randomized controlled Trial in Bihar, India. *Journal of global health.* Dec 2019;9(2):0204249. doi:10.7189/jogh.09.020424

55.   Carmichael SL, Mehta K, Raheel H, et al. Effects of team-based goals and non-monetary incentives on front-line health worker performance and maternal health behaviours: a cluster randomised controlled trial in Bihar, India. *BMJ Glob Health.* 2019;4(4):e001146. doi:10.1136/bmjgh-2018-001146

56.   Grant C, Nawal D, Guntur SM, et al. 'We pledge to improve the health of our entire community': Improving health worker motivation and performance in Bihar, India through teamwork, recognition, and non-financial incentives. *PLoS One.* 2018;13(8):e0203265. doi:10.1371/journal.pone.0203265

57.   Das A, Nawal D, Singh MK, et al. Impact of a Nursing Skill-Improvement Intervention on Newborn-Specific Delivery Practices: An Experience from Bihar, India. *Birth.* Dec 2016;43(4):328-335. doi:10.1111/birt.12239

58.   Das A, Nawal D, Singh MK, et al. Evaluation of the mobile nurse training (MNT) intervention - a step towards improvement in intrapartum practices in Bihar, India. *BMC Pregnancy Childbirth.* Aug 23 2017;17(1):266. doi:10.1186/s12884-017-1452-z

59.   National Health Mission, Ministry of Health & Family Welfare, Government of India. Reproductive, Maternal, Newborn, Child and Adolescent Health (RMNCH+A). GoI. April 22, 2020. Accessed April 22, 2020. https://nhm.gov.in/index1.php?lang=1&level=1&sublinkid=794&lid=168

60.   Ministry of Health & Family Welfare, Government of India. A strategic approach to Reproductive, Maternal, Newborn, Child and Adolescent health (RMNCH+A) in India. Govt. of India; 2013. http://cghealth.nic.in/nhmcg/Informations/RMNCH/1_RMNCHA_Strategy.pdf

61.   Maternal and Child Health Integrated Program (MCHIP), USAID. *India's Reproductive, Maternal, Newborn, Child, and Adolescent Health (RMNCH+A) Strategy*. 2014. Accessed April 21, 2020. https://www.mchip.net/sites/default/files/RMNCH+A%20in%20India.pdf

62.   Government of Bihar. Bihar Vikas Mission: Human Development Sub-Mission GoB. April 22, 2020. Accessed April 22, 2020. https://www.bvm.bihar.gov.in/content/3752/humandevelopmentsubmission

63.   Creanga AA, Srikantiah S, Mahapatra T, et al. Statewide implementation of a quality improvement initiative for reproductive, maternal, newborn and child health and nutritionin Bihar, India. *Journal of global health*. Dec 2020;10(2):021008. doi:10.7189/jogh.10.021008

64.   Govt. of Bihar. Bihar Medical Services & Infrastructure Corporation Limited. Department of Health and Family Welfare. March 25, 2020. Accessed March 25, , 2020. http://bmsicl.gov.in/

65.   CARE India. Strengthening Supply Chain of Essential Medicines Through E Aushadhi Intervention. CARE India. April 23, 2020. Accessed April 23, 2020. https://www.careindia.org/bihar/case_studies/streamlining_of_fp_supply_chain.html

66.   CARE India. Strengthening and Streamlining of FP Supply Chain through FPLMIS. CARE India. April 23, 2020. Accessed April 23, 2020. https://www.careindia.org/bihar/case_studies/e_aushadhi.html

67.   CARE India. A model for mentorship: Mobile Nurse Mentoring. *Resources and Publications: Health.* CARE India; 2018. 2018. April 20, 2020. https://www.careindia.org/wp-content/uploads/2019/07/Bihar_4_REV_SCREEN.pdf

68.   Ghosh R, Spindler H, Morgan MC, et al. Diagnosis and management of postpartum hemorrhage and intrapartum asphyxia in a quality improvement initiative using nurse-mentoring and simulation in Bihar, India. *PLoS One.* 2019;14(7):e0216654. doi:10.1371/journal.pone.0216654

69.   Raney JH, Morgan MC, Christmas A, et al. Simulation-enhanced nurse mentoring to improve preeclampsia and eclampsia care: an education intervention study in Bihar, India. *BMC Pregnancy Childbirth.* Jan 23 2019;19(1):41. doi:10.1186/s12884-019-2186-x

70.   Ahmed S, Srivastava S, Warren N, et al. The impact of a nurse mentoring program on the quality of labour and delivery care at primary health care facilities in Bihar, India. *BMJ Glob Health.* 2019;4(6):e001767. doi:10.1136/bmjgh-2019-001767

71.   CARE India. Health System Progress Tracker Dashboard. CARE India. April 23, 2020. Accessed April 23, 2020. https://www.careindia.org/bihar/case_studies/health_system_progress_tracker.html#

72.   CARE India. Darpan Plus Supervision ICT. CARE India. April 23, 2020. Accessed April 23, 2020. https://www.careindia.org/bihar/case_studies/darpan_plus_supervision.html

73.   Bihar State Health Society. Darpan Classic. Govt. of Bihar. April 23, 2020. Accessed April 23, 2020. http://bi.careindia.org:8030/fro/submissionstatus

74.	Knaul FM, Bhadelia A, Atun R, Frenk J. Achieving Effective Universal Health Coverage And Diagonal Approaches To Care For Chronic Illnesses. *Health Aff (Millwood)*. Sep 2015;34(9):1514-22. doi:10.1377/hlthaff.2015.0514

75.	Assefa Y, Tesfaye D, Damme WV, Hill PS. Effectiveness and sustainability of a diagonal investment approach to strengthen the primary health-care system in Ethiopia. *Lancet*. Oct 20 2018;392(10156):1473-1481. doi:10.1016/s0140-6736(18)32215-3

76.	Government of India. *Bihar: Road map for development of health sector - a report of the Special Task Force on Bihar*. 20017. Accessed Febriary 20, 2020. http://164.100.161.239/aboutus/taskforce/tsk_bhs.pdf

77.	World Health Organization. Everybody's Business: Strengthening health systems to improve health outcomes - WHO's framework for action. WHO Press; 2007:56. https://www.who.int/healthsystems/strategy/everybodys_business.pdf

78.	Patel R, Ladusingh L. Do Physical Proximity and Availability of Adequate Infrastructure at Public Health Facility Increase Institutional Delivery? A Three Level Hierarchical Model Approach. *PLoS One*. 2015;10(12):e0144352. doi:10.1371/journal.pone.0144352

79.	McFadden A, Gupta S, Marshall JL, et al. Systematic review of barriers to, and facilitators of, the provision of high-quality midwifery services in India. *Birth*. Jul 25 2020;doi:10.1111/birt.12498

80.	Jimenez Soto E, La Vincente S, Clark A, et al. Investment case for improving maternal and child health: results from four countries. *BMC Public Health*. 2013;13:601. doi:1471-2458-13-601 [pii]
10.1186/1471-2458-13-601 [doi]

81.   Singh A. Shortage and inequalities in the distribution of specialists across community health centres in Uttar Pradesh, 2002-2012. *BMC health services research*. May 24 2019;19(1):331. doi:10.1186/s12913-019-4134-x

82.   Hanson C, Singh S, Zamboni K, et al. Care practices and neonatal survival in 52 neonatal intensive care units in Telangana and Andhra Pradesh, India: A cross-sectional study. *PLoS medicine*. Jul 2019;16(7):e1002860. doi:10.1371/journal.pmed.1002860

83.   Karan A, Negandhi H, Nair R, Sharma A, Tiwari R, Zodpey S. Size, composition and distribution of human resource for health in India: new estimates using National Sample Survey and Registry data. *BMJ Open*. May 27 2019;9(4):e025979. doi:10.1136/bmjopen-2018-025979

84.   Pakhare A, Kumar S, Goyal S, Joshi R. Assessment of primary care facilities for cardiovascular disease preparedness in Madhya Pradesh, India. *BMC health services research*. Sep 23 2015;15:408. doi:10.1186/s12913-015-1075-x

85.   Taneja G, Sridhar VS, Mohanty JS, et al. India's RMNCH+A Strategy: approach, learnings and limitations. *BMJ Glob Health*. 2019;4(3):e001162. doi:10.1136/bmjgh-2018-001162

86.   Department of Health and Family Welfare, Ministry of Health and Family Welfare, Govt of India. List of High Priority Districts identified by the department of Health and Family Welfare. Govt. of India. December 27, 2020. Accessed December 27, 2020. https://data.gov.in/catalog/list-high-priority-districts-identified-department-health-and-family-welfare?filters%5Bfield_catalog_reference%5D=95958&format=json&offset=0&limit=6&sort%5Bcreated%5D=desc

87.   Dobility, Inc. SurveyCTO. May 5, 2021. Accessed May 5, 2021. https://www.surveycto.com/

88.	The Open Data Kit (ODK) Project. Open Data Kit. March 25, 2019. Accessed March 25, 2019. https://opendatakit.org/

89.	National Health Mission, Govt. of India. 5x5 Matrix for High Impact RMNCH+A Interventions Govt. of India; 2014. December 27, 2020. Accessed December 27, 2020. https://nhm.gov.in/images/pdf/programmes/maternal-health/guidelines/5x5_matrix_2502.pdf

90.	Kc A, Singh DR, Upadhyaya MK, Budhathoki SS, Gurung A, Målqvist M. Quality of Care for Maternal and Newborn Health in Health Facilities in Nepal. *Matern Child Health J*. Feb 2020;24(Suppl 1):31-38. doi:10.1007/s10995-019-02846-w

91.	Tomlin K, Berhanu D, Gautham M, et al. Assessing capacity of health facilities to provide routine maternal and newborn care in low-income settings: what proportions are ready to provide good-quality care, and what proportions of women receive it? *BMC Pregnancy Childbirth*. May 12 2020;20(1):289. doi:10.1186/s12884-020-02926-8

92.	Gabrysch S, Civitelli G, Edmond KM, et al. New signal functions to measure the ability of health facilities to provide routine and emergency newborn care. *PLoS medicine*. 2012;9(11):e1001340. doi:10.1371/journal.pmed.1001340

93.	Vesel L, Manu A, Lohela TJ, et al. Quality of newborn care: a health facility assessment in rural Ghana using survey, vignette and surveillance data. *BMJ Open*. May 9 2013;3(5)doi:10.1136/bmjopen-2012-002326

94.	WHO, UNICEF. *Water, sanitation and hygiene in health care facilities Status in low- and middle-income countries and way forward*. 2015. Accessed February 20, 2020. https://apps.who.int/iris/bitstream/handle/10665/154588/9789241508476_eng.pdf;jsessionid=E451186F2CA3F2144BB8D0B0EC9F3859?sequence=1

95.   Kozuki N, Oseni L, Mtimuni A, et al. Health facility service availability and readiness for intrapartum and immediate postpartum care in Malawi: A cross-sectional survey. *PLoS One.* 2017;12(3):e0172492. doi:10.1371/journal.pone.0172492

96.   Lama TP, Munos MK, Katz J, Khatry SK, LeClerq SC, Mullany LC. Assessment of facility and health worker readiness to provide quality antenatal, intrapartum and postpartum care in rural Southern Nepal. *BMC health services research.* Jan 6 2020;20(1):16. doi:10.1186/s12913-019-4871-x

97.   Winter R, Yourkavitch J, Wang W, Mallick L. Assessment of health facility capacity to provide newborn care in Bangladesh, Haiti, Malawi, Senegal, and Tanzania. *Journal of global health.* Dec 2017;7(2):020509. doi:10.7189/jogh.07.020509

98.   Federal Ministry of Health Ethiopia, UNFPA. *National Health Facility Assessment on Reproductive Health Commodities and Services in Ethiopia 2015.* 2015. Accessed December 20, 2020. https://ethiopia.unfpa.org/en/resources/national-health-facility-assessment-reproductive-health-commodities-and-services-ethiopia

99.   Ekenna A, Itanyi IU, Nwokoro U, Hirschhorn LR, Uzochukwu B. How ready is the system to deliver primary healthcare? Results of a primary health facility assessment in Enugu State, Nigeria. *Health Policy Plan.* Nov 1 2020;35(Supplement_1):i97-i106. doi:10.1093/heapol/czaa108

100.   Bintabara D, Ernest A, Mpondo B. Health facility service availability and readiness to provide basic emergency obstetric and newborn care in a low-resource setting: evidence from a Tanzania National Survey. *BMJ Open.* Feb 19 2019;9(2):e020608. doi:10.1136/bmjopen-2017-020608

101.   Powell-Jackson T, Acharya A, Mills A. An assessment of the quality of primary health care in India. *Econ Polit Wkly*. 2013;48(19):53–61.

102.   Ethiopian Public Health Institute, Federal Ministry of Health Ethiopia. *Ethiopia Service Availability and Readiness Assessment (SARA) 2018 Final Report* 2018. May, 2018. Accessed December 20, 2020. https://www.ephi.gov.et/images/pictures/download_2011/Ethiopia-Service-Availability-and-Rediness-Assessment-SARA-report-2018.pdf

103.   Abdalla S, Weng Y, Mehta KM, et al. Trends in reproductive, maternal, newborn and child health and nutrition indicators during five years of piloting and scaling-up of Ananya interventions in Bihar, India. *Journal of global health*. Dec 2020;10(2):021003. doi:10.7189/jogh.10.021003

104.   Olivier de Sardan JP, Diarra A, Koné FY, Yaogo M, Zerbo R. Local sustainability and scaling up for user fee exemptions: medical NGOs vis-à-vis health systems. *BMC health services research*. 2015;15 Suppl 3(Suppl 3):S5. doi:10.1186/1472-6963-15-s3-s5

105.   Pfeiffer J, Johnson W, Fort M, et al. Strengthening health systems in poor countries: a code of conduct for nongovernmental organizations. *Am J Public Health*. Dec 2008;98(12):2134-40. doi:10.2105/ajph.2007.125989

106.   Health Statistics and Information Systems, World Health Organization. *Service Availability and Readiness Assessment (SARA): an annual monitoring system for service delivery Reference Manual, Version 2.2*. 2015. Accessed October 30, 2020. https://www.who.int/healthinfo/systems/sara_reference_manual/en/

107.   Nambiar D, Sankar H, Negi J, Nair A, Sadanandan R. Field-testing of primary health-care indicators, India. *Bull World Health Organ*. 2020;98(11):747–753. doi:10.2471/BLT.19.249565

108.   Nambiar D, Sankar DH, Negi J, Nair A, Sadanandan R. Monitoring Universal Health Coverage reforms in primary health care facilities: Creating a framework, selecting and field-testing indicators in Kerala, India. *PLoS One*. 2020;15(8):e0236169. doi:10.1371/journal.pone.0236169

109.   WHO, UNAIDS, PEPFAR. *Task shifting : rational redistribution of tasks among health workforce teams : global recommendations and guidelines.* 2008. https://www.who.int/healthsystems/TTR-TaskShifting.pdf?ua=1

110.   European Commission. *TASK SHIFTING AND HEALTH SYSTEM DESIGN: Report of the Expert Panel on effective ways of investing in Health (EXPH).* 2019. Accessed August 8, 2021. https://ec.europa.eu/health/sites/default/files/expert_panel/docs/023_taskshifting_en.pdf

111.   Spindler H, Dyer J, Bagchi K, et al. Tracking and debriefing birth data at scale: A mobile phone application to improve obstetric and neonatal care in Bihar, India. *Nurs Open*. Jul 2018;5(3):267-274. doi:10.1002/nop2.134

112.   Higgins BV, Medvedev MM, Spindler H, et al. Cohort study of neonatal resuscitation skill retention in frontline healthcare facilities in Bihar, India, after PRONTO simulation training. *BMJ Paediatr Open*. 2020;4(1):e000628. doi:10.1136/bmjpo-2019-000628

113.   Blanc AK, Diaz C, McCarthy KJ, Berdichevsky K. Measuring progress in maternal and newborn health care in Mexico: validating indicators of health system contact and quality of care. *BMC Pregnancy Childbirth*. Aug 30 2016;16(1):255. doi:10.1186/s12884-016-1047-0

114.   Nesbitt RC, Lohela TJ, Manu A, et al. Quality along the continuum: a health facility assessment of intrapartum and postnatal care in Ghana. *PLoS One*. 2013;8(11):e81089. doi:10.1371/journal.pone.0081089

115.   Bedoya G, Dolinger A, Rogo K, et al. Observations of infection prevention and control practices in primary health care, Kenya. *Bull World Health Organ*. Jul 1 2017;95(7):503-516. doi:10.2471/blt.16.179499

116.   de Graft-Johnson J, Vesel L, Rosen HE, et al. Cross-sectional observational assessment of quality of newborn care immediately after birth in health facilities across six sub-Saharan African countries. *BMJ Open*. Mar 27 2017;7(3):e014680. doi:10.1136/bmjopen-2016-014680

117.   Leslie HH, Sun Z, Kruk ME. Association between infrastructure and observed quality of care in 4 healthcare services: A cross-sectional study of 4,300 facilities in 8 countries. *PLoS medicine*. Dec 2017;14(12):e1002464. doi:10.1371/journal.pmed.1002464

118.   Kaur J, Franzen SRP, Newton-Lewis T, Murphy G. Readiness of public health facilities to provide quality maternal and newborn care across the state of Bihar, India: a cross-sectional study of district hospitals and primary health centres. *BMJ Open*. Jul 29 2019;9(7):e028370. doi:10.1136/bmjopen-2018-028370

119.   Vail B, Morgan MC, Dyer J, et al. Logistical, cultural, and structural barriers to immediate neonatal care and neonatal resuscitation in Bihar, India. *BMC Pregnancy Childbirth*. Sep 29 2018;18(1):385. doi:10.1186/s12884-018-2017-5

120.   Morgan MC, Dyer J, Abril A, et al. Barriers and facilitators to the provision of optimal obstetric and neonatal emergency care and to the implementation of simulation-enhanced mentorship in primary care facilities in Bihar, India: a qualitative study. *BMC Pregnancy Childbirth*. Oct 25 2018;18(1):420. doi:10.1186/s12884-018-2059-8

121.   Lohela TJ, Nesbitt RC, Manu A, et al. Competence of health workers in emergency obstetric care: an assessment using clinical vignettes in Brong Ahafo region, Ghana. *BMJ Open*. Jun 13 2016;6(6):e010963. doi:10.1136/bmjopen-2015-010963

122. Ueno E, Adegoke AA, Masenga G, Fimbo J, Msuya SE. Skilled birth attendants in Tanzania: a descriptive study of cadres and emergency obstetric care signal functions performed. *Matern Child Health J*. Jan 2015;19(1):155-69. doi:10.1007/s10995-014-1506-z

123. Helfinstein S, Jain M, Ramesh BM, et al. Facilities are substantially more influential than care providers in the quality of delivery care received: a variance decomposition and clustering analysis in Kenya, Malawi and India. *BMJ Glob Health*. Aug 2020;5(8)doi:10.1136/bmjgh-2020-002437

124. World Health Organization. Promoting baby-friendly hospitals. WHO. August 13, 2021. Accessed August 13, 2021. https://www.who.int/activities/promoting-baby-friendly-hospitals

www.ingramcontent.com/pod-product-compliance
Lightning Source LLC
LaVergne TN
LVHW040013200726
843493LV00005B/1243